Between You and Me

Between You and Me:

A Sensible and Authoritative Guide to the Care and Treatment of your Skin

John A. Parrish, M.D.
Barbara A. Gilchrest, M.D.
Thomas B. Fitzpatrick, M.D.

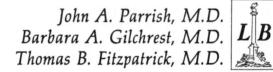

Little, Brown and Company   *Boston–Toronto*

First Edition

T 10/78

The illustration on page 168 is from *Plant Toxicity and Dermatitis: A
Manual for Physicians* by Kenneth F. Lampe. Copyright © 1968 by The
Williams & Wilkins Co., Baltimore Md.

Library of Congress Cataloging in Publication Data

Parrish, John Albert, 1939–
    Between you and me.

    Includes index.
    1. Skin—Care and hygiene. I. Gilchrest,
Barbara A., joint author. II. Fitzpatrick, Thomas B.,
joint author. III. Title.
RL87.P37   616.5'05   78-16592
ISBN 0-316-69252-2

Designed by Janis Capone

*Published simultaneously in Canada by Little, Brown & Company (Canada)
Limited*

PRINTED IN THE UNITED STATES OF AMERICA

Contents

Acknowledgments

Although this approach to communicating with our patients about the skin and its problems is our own, we have had the help of many persons in the writing of this book. The concepts discussed in the first three chapters are influenced by the writing of Ashley Montagu (*Touching: The Human Significance of the Skin*, New York: Columbia University Press, 1971), Weston La-Barre (*The Human Animal*, University of Chicago Press, 1955), several books by Ernest Becker (especially *The Structure of Evil*, New York: The Free Press, 1968), and by the teachings and writings of Dr. Theodore Nadelson. Dr. Irvin H. Blank offered helpful criticisms of the entire book and specific contributions to Chapters 4 and 7. Consideration of the microenvironment of the skin from the point of view of microbes was suggested to us by the artistic prose of Theodor Rosebury and Dr. Albert Kligman and Dr. M. J. Marples.

We are grateful for creative criticism of the manuscript by Joan Parrish, Byron Gilchrest, Joe Merman, Dr. Kathleen O'Shea, and especially thankful for the review, editing, and alterations by Bea Fitzpatrick. Mr. Llewellyn Howland and Mr. Richard P. McDonough of

Little, Brown and Company provided helpful direction and assistance and expert editorial advice. The manuscript was typed and retyped by Wendy Fong.

Our greatest debt is to our patients. They challenge us and teach us.

Acknowledgments

Preface

You have not been given a square deal in the management of your skin problems. Because skin diseases are seldom medical emergencies or mortal illnesses, the dissemination of misinformation and ineffective therapy by druggists, friends, and even physicians has been condoned. The fact remains, however, that skin diseases account for a large percentage of medical complaints, are usually benign but not necessarily so, and continue to have a major impact—social and psychological—on their victims.

Times are changing. In the past, physicians were considered the proper repository of all medical knowledge. Patients were told as little as possible about the nature of their illnesses and medications. People who could not afford to see a physician learned nothing about these subjects. Today most physicians acknowledge the right of patients to know the diagnosis, the etiology of the ailment, what its possible repercussions might be, and what treatment options exist. Unfortunately, limitations of time often drastically compromise the transfer of this information. A busy doctor cannot answer all of the patient's questions, even if the patient is prepared to ask them. Doctors often do not encourage questions. This is not necessarily bad will on the part of physicians—it is a fact of medical economics. The real tragedy is that good medical advice is nearly impossible to find in another setting. This is especially true in the area of dermatology. Even the carefully researched and well-intentioned dermatologic articles that appear by the score in newspapers and magazines are too often wrong. Dermatologists are by far the most reliable source of such information but seem bound by tradition and unspoken taboos from disseminating it except in the one-to-one, doctor-patient setting. Despite the obvious need for better public health education, only a handful of physicians in any specialty risk peer disapproval to share their knowledge through books, radio and television programs, and other forms of mass media.

How much has been learned in recent years about both common and exotic skin diseases! For many disorders, previously haphazard remedies have evolved into medically sound, effective treatments. The public needs and deserves ready access to this knowledge.

There are no secrets in medicine. You may hear about Dr. Smith's or Ms. Jones's new "miracle" cures for aging, acne, psoriasis, baldness, or a variety of other skin problems. But any truly effective new therapy rapidly becomes known to physicians around the world and thus is available to all patients.

Our subject is common skin problems, readily identified by most people with or without a medical background, and personally familiar to all too many of us. This book is not a guide to self-diagnosis. Pictures of skin lesions and detailed written descriptions have been omitted largely to discourage "matching up" an unknown skin lesion with an entity in the book. Such guesswork is exceedingly dangerous. This book may complement a visit to the doctor but does not replace it.

The "inactive" ingredients in many creams and ointments may be as critical to successful therapy as the "medicine" they contain. Hence, in this book we recommend certain products by brand name because we have found these specific preparations to be helpful. Undoubtedly, equally effective products have been omitted.

Through the book, we hope to provide some help for people with skin disorders, to correct certain common misconceptions, and to share our interest in this truly remarkable organ—our skin.

I

AN
OVERVIEW OF
THE SKIN

1
The
Concept
of Beauty

When we present our clothed bodies to the world, the visible 5 percent of our skin surface is one gauge of acceptance or rejection that strongly influences how people react to us. We carefully examine the skin and facial features of persons in forming a first impression. We tend to estimate intelligence, social status, sexual appeal, and power at least partly on the exposed surfaces of the face, neck, and hands. We form preliminary opinions: respect, admiration, desire, disgust. We often subconsciously predict the outcome of a dominance struggle and decide if we are threatened. We make hundreds of these judgments daily. Instantly. Automatically.

As we scan the populace, people may come to our attention if they satisfy or jar our sense of beauty. Now, as throughout history, the contours, texture, and color of one's skin have great psychic impact and strongly influence the chances of achieving material, sexual, and social satisfaction. The complexion, color, and contour that conform with class norms can impart automatic high status in the relative absence of other personal attributes. On the other hand, harmless variations in pigmentation, gland function, or hair growth can lead to complete ostracism. People have been worshiped as gods or sentenced to lifelong slavery depending on the amount of pigment in the skin.

We take skin aesthetics seriously. We exaggerate, modify, or diminish naturally occurring skin colors, gland excretions, and hair. The cosmetic industry reinforces, stimulates, and sometimes creates the need to make specific alterations in the appearance, texture, and smell of our skin. Most people apply at least one chemical daily to alter their skin. Even the most liberated women continue to paint or pluck some part of their faces. We seek to modify our bodies to achieve a complicated aesthetic image. We wish to enhance sexuality, youth, and ethnic and racial ideals. We try to change that which is not consistent with our concept of beauty, a concept determined by complicated sociological, geographical, and historical factors.

Our aesthetic self-awareness is simply a statement of our humanity. One aspect is the denial of animal biology. We must clearly separate ourselves from other mammals. We deny our animal nature by our grooming habits, by removing and cutting hair, and by trimming nails. We do not want to smell our bodies, and so we keep all body orifices scrupulously clean and sweetly scented.

We even aspire to immortality. Our aesthetic judgment is shaped and colored by this yearning. The beautiful is that which has transcendent qualities. The beautiful is that which is potential, germinative, involuntary, uncaused — Alpha. The ugly is actualized, materialized, fabricated, caused — Omega. The yearning for immortality fashions an aesthetic sense that embraces youth, sexuality, and ethnocentricity. Youth is

4

the new, the beginning, the fresh. Youthful skin also has appeal to us through memory and association. In our infancy the skin was a source of great sensual satisfaction. From the time our brain cells, nerve cells, and skin cells first connected in the early weeks of uterine life until the time of weaning, the skin was the mediator for the most intense, warm and dependent relationship we would ever encounter. From this vantage point, we were loved completely and unconditionally. We received affirmation of that love through touches and caresses and tender soothing skin care.

Desire for youthful appearance of skin is also an expression of our fear of aging, our denial of death, and our subsequent low esteem of the aged. We insist that youth itself is beautiful. Our sense of beauty requires skin like a baby's: smooth, flawless, unwrinkled, relatively hairless, uniform in color, and soft. The normal biologic changes that occur in the skin as the result of maturing and aging are undesirable. Unlike John Donne, we see no beauty in an "autumnal face." The thin, dull, gray hair and the dry, scaly skin of the aged are not considered badges of respectable seniority. They are viewed as ugly. We are repulsed by pale and blotchy skin that has a parchmentlike texture. Wrinkling and dryness remind us of death itself.

In an attempt to re-create infantile skin, we remove hair that is part of the maturation process. Men shave their faces, women shave legs and armpits and pluck facial hair. Creams and lotions soften the skin. To combat wrinkling, the most obvious sign of age, people even sometimes resort to surgery.

Beauty is often equated with sexuality. The skin is one expression of sexuality. The texture and the distribution of hair and fat display maleness or femaleness.

5

Many of the glands of the skin are sensitive to sex hormones and begin to function at puberty. Skin also responds to the sex hormones to advertise pregnancy by changing blood flow and pigment distribution. The skin can be considered a sex organ; it receives and transmits the intimate messages of arousal and changes its blood flow during sexual excitement.

We make judgments about sexual appeal rapidly and subliminally, and we make them constantly. The nonseasonal sexual receptivity of the human female not only creates and fulfills a requirement for family life but also gives sex the potential to occupy a part of our thought and action at all times. And should our instinctual capacity for sexual thought ever diminish, the advertising business will quickly restimulate us.

All human desires and concerns shape our aesthetic concepts. Beauty is what we want, tempered by what we are. We want to be part of a group. We are part of a group. The prolonged dependent state of *Homo sapiens* is cause, effect, and correlate of the development of a desire for affiliation. In order to transcend his animal nature, man desired identification, loyalty, investment, and absorption into a group that outnumbered and outlived him. Eventually family ties evolved into tribal loyalties. The tendency to affiliate, cooperate, and form units later produced societies. Selective inbreeding and genetic drifts led to development of characteristic physical features for each subgroup of the human population.

The drive for affiliation influenced the sense of beauty. The sense of beauty, in turn, influenced and molded the group through its effect on mate selection. Although the concept of physical beauty varies from person to person, there is, among defined groups of

6

persons, a striking unanimity about who and what is beautiful. The features that any one group selects to admire are usually those that most typify the ideal of that group. Sense of beauty came to be familial, then tribal, then ethnocentric, and, at times, nationalistic. Emulation of certain features enhances a person's sense of belonging. At the same time, group labeling and loyalty create a mechanism for projecting undesirable human qualities onto people clearly identified as outside of the group, people with different physical features.

Compared to the slow, simplistic Darwinian concept of evolution based on qualities necessary for survival, the genetic grouping of features compatible with racial and ethnic sense of beauty is variable, arbitrary, and biologically trivial. As a cosmetic creature, man confounds evolution.

Beauty is, in a partial sense, the approximation of a racial or ethnic norm. We tend to "beautify" ourselves by emphasizing the traits that typify our group. The naturally pink cheeks of Caucasoid women are painted pinker and red lips made redder. White skin is made whiter cosmetically. If blond hair is idealized, it is achieved chemically. Hair is made wavy or straight or frizzy to accent and magnify racial norms. At times beautification is carried to the extremes of mutilating or altering body contours. Big lips of the Ubangis are stretched and made bigger, small feet of Oriental women are bound and made smaller, relatively hairless American Indians remove what hair remains.

Marketing and advertising professionals convince us that their cosmetics, soaps, and vitamins help us achieve all of the elusive ideals. "Hate that gray; wash it away!" "Look like a bride again!" "Which is the

7

daughter and which is the mother?" "Your moist lips are more kissable." "This shampoo leaves your hair manageable" (orderly and uniform like a good human being), "vibrant and full" (youthful), "straight" (Caucasoid), "curly" (Negroid), "lusty, flowing with body" (sexy as hell).

We may applaud or deplore the rationale for our aesthetic sense, but we cannot deny the importance of this obsession in our daily lives. Of course, beauty involves not only the physical. As Sir James Barrie put it in *What Every Woman Knows:*

Alick: What is charm, exactly, Maggie?
Maggie: Oh, it's . . . it's a sort of bloom on a woman. If you have it, you don't need to have anything else; and if you don't have it, it doesn't matter what else you have.

However, as long as a youthful, healthy appearance remains central to our image of beauty, we will need to concentrate on the skin, that most sensitive indicator of both age and illness. We must learn how to maintain healthy, youthful-appearing skin, to recognize the common skin diseases and to master their prevention or treatment, and to sort dermatologic fact from fiction.

The Concept of Beauty

2

Psychological
Importance
of Skin

Skin is anatomically and symbolically involved in man's most basic idea of himself and his world. Skin is the boundary between the inside and the outside, between the self and non-self. Attitudes, prejudices, and symbols about skin stem from man's fundamental views of his own life and purpose.

The infant's primitive perception of the world is a jumble of impulses, sensations, and experiences that do not clearly separate the infant self from the world about him. Images and light appear and disappear. Sensations come and go. The infant has no way of knowing whether a sensation is a corporate part of his being or a passing object of no importance. When a sensation ceases, the infant does not know whether its cause is dead and gone or temporarily withdrawn but still a part of a real and tangible world. Cries control the mother, who touches and withdraws, and may or may not be an extension of the infant body. There is no clear separation of the world into self and non-self.

As the brain matures, we learn to compartmentalize the world: the real and unreal, the tangible and the abstract, the self and non-self. The skin is actually and

9

symbolically the boundary between self and non-self. Maintaining the integrity of the skin maintains the separation.

But self and non-self is only the first dualism we accept as we expand our view of ourselves. The ability to conceptualize the past, present, and future leads to our basic predicament. We realize that we are biologic animals with a life cycle, physical needs, and certain death; but at the same time we know ourselves to be ethereal schemers and dreamers capable of eternal thoughts, transcendent ideas, and immortal desires. The comparison may cause us to resent or deny the animal part of our nature, but we are bound by biologic laws and physical needs. Thoughts can take us anywhere, but we are limited by our bodies. We pursue salvation in that which is mental, that which is heavenly, that which is within others, that which is beyond the body — beyond the boundaries of our own skin. Again, the skin symbolizes a boundary, a separation, a limit.

We wish to deny the biologic animal — that which is within. This denial is so strong that we actually learn to be repulsed by our insides. It is our animal, limited, physical self. Our feces is solid waste that reminds us of animality, decay, and death. We are taught to be sickened by its smell, appearance, and consistency. Urine is a body waste. When products are allowed to leave the inside of our body, their exit must be quickly and efficiently achieved in private and then they must quickly be put out of sight.

That which is inside should remain inside or at least not be brought to our attention. Food in the stomach is in the process of being incorporated. It should be kept within. Vomitus, food mixed with body fluids, disgusts

10

us. To spit at another person is to defile him. Exposure of blood or viscera makes us faint.

Learning to keep the inside contained or to expel it efficiently in private is a part of the socialization process. We learn to control the natural spontaneous expulsion of body wastes. We learn not to explore the body orifices or to be curious about their contents. We develop a body control that keeps our insides under wraps. Using the weapon of shame, our parents teach us to guard against our insides ever breaking out. We fear revealing anything that should be hidden.

The inside of our body is over 70 percent water. Everything within is wet. Blood, urine, and vomitus are liquid. The skin that surrounds entrances to the wet inner body is moist, and the outer surface of the body is dry. Inside is wet, outside is dry. The skin is the boundary.

The symbolic importance of skin becomes more obvious when we examine attitudes toward skin disease. A lesion on the skin is an insult to our aesthetic sense, an imperfection. But the lesion also interrupts the physical integrity of the skin and threatens our separation of self and non-self. Worst of all, the lesion is a repulsive exposure of our inner self: body fluids, or the redness of blood. Our compulsive attempt to keep our insides stifled is foiled. That which should be on the inside is on the outside. It is unclean and wet. We remember our early training and are ashamed.

A single pimple on the forehead causes great embarrassment even though we know it is not dangerous, does not signify systemic disease, and is not contagious. Why? Because it is an escape of the inside. We speak of rashes as "breaking out." All "breakings out" of our insides are a source of shame. A stigma. We feel responsible and somehow guilty that such a thing is possible.

The concept of contagion magnifies the shame and embarrassment caused by skin disease. We all know that some types of skin lesions may be spread to others by touching. Persons with certain infections of the skin should be avoided. They should not be touched. The emotional attitude toward untouchable skin disease becomes generalized to include common noncontagious skin lesions. Not too long ago, in a large hospital in Vienna, all dermatology patients were relegated to the psychiatric wards to share quarters with victims of other "shameful" diseases.

It is no wonder that people with skin disease often have a "leper complex." They are ashamed that their insides are unmasked; they are threatened by the loss of the physical integrity of their skin. They feel as though they may cause spread of disease to others. They feel something may be seriously wrong with them. At the same time, they are reminded of their animality.

These are some of the reasons we feel embarrassed when we have skin lesions. Most often the shame is not based on the facts relating to the contagion, loss of function, or symptoms of a rash, but on the complex psychological factors that determine our attitudes toward the skin. It is most likely that many of those labeled as pariahs and "untouchables" in biblical times did not have leprosy or any other infectious disease. Close examination of ancient records suggests that they had harmless pigment disorders, psoriasis, and eczema. Their forced isolation was not due to the possibility of contagion but to their own guilt and the attitude of their fellowmen.

12

3

Communication
through the Skin

Humans can survive without vision, hearing, smell, or taste, but they cannot survive without the sensory functions of the skin. We communicate with the world through our skin. Messages are received and transmitted constantly. These communications are necessary for our comfort. They are also a prerequisite of life. Cutaneous sensory input is also necessary for emotional maturation and psychological stability.

The skin arises from the ectoderm, outermost of the three embryonic cell layers. The ectoderm is the source of the other sense organs, which survey and analyze the environment by smell, vision, taste, and hearing. The ectoderm also gives rise to the nervous system.

The sense of touch is the earliest of the senses to develop in the human, being present when the embryo is less than one inch long. The microscopic nerve fibers that conduct touch impulses from the skin to the brain generally develop earliest *in utero* and become larger than other peripheral nerves. Man's sensitive skin receives tremendous numbers of impulses that must be organized and transmitted to the spinal cord and brain. Because man is such a large, relatively naked, and

13

sensitive animal, a large part of the brain must be designated to assimilate and react to skin messages. Some of these impulses are transmitted to conscious thinking and many more are automatically acted upon without our being aware of them.

Through its hairs, its vast network of nerves, and its specialized sensory receptors, our skin provides a sophisticated sensor to inform us about our world. Pain. Pressure. Temperature. Data about things touching the skin are accumulated and synthesized in the brain: consistency, shape, texture, temperature, and weight. We learn who or what is touching us.

To keep us aware of our environment is one aspect of the skin's fundamental role of protection. We do not have the hard shell of an armadillo. Because we have more behavioral options than the armadillo, we need a more refined form of communication with our environment and can compensate for a frailer physical barrier. We are covered by a complicated sensor that can initiate reactions in our bodies and can itself react. The skin not only senses changes in ambient temperature but makes automatic adjustments in blood flow and perspiration rate to adjust the body temperature. The skin protects us by notifying us of noxious stimuli, excess pressure, blunt or sharp trauma, and other environmental insults. Conscious and unconscious body shifts and adjustments can then be made to avoid cuts, burns, and pressure sores. Absence of pain fibers in the skin quickly leads to repeated trauma, ulceration, and the death of tissue.

The ability of the skin to detect sensation not only provides understanding about our environment and protection from potentially harmful elements, it also provides us with pleasure and a means for communi-
14   cation with others. Such communication actually nur-

tures the physical and behavioral growth and development of man. Studies of lower animals have shown that licking, stroking, grooming, and cuddling are essential to normal development of the young. In fact, some newborn animals do not survive unless licked or groomed by their mothers soon after birth, even if such attention is not necessary to clear breathing passages. Cutaneous stimulation may be necessary to normal development of the autonomic nervous system, which controls respiration and other vital activities. Tender loving care in the form of touching is similarly essential to the physical and emotional survival of the human infant. "It is the handling, the carrying, the caressing, and the cuddling that we would here emphasize," writes Ashley Montagu, "for it would seem that even in the absence of a great deal else, these are the reassuringly basic experiences the infant must enjoy if it is to survive in some semblance of health. Extreme sensory deprivation in other respects, such as light and sound, can be survived as long as the sensory experiences at the skin are maintained."*

Humans cover themselves with clothing from infancy. This tends to reduce the number and extent of pleasurable sensations from the skin. Actual or symbolic shedding of clothing may represent attempts to regain some of this blunted sensual experience and may explain the nonsexual joy that nudists claim to experience from the feel of the wind, air, and sun upon the body.

Later in life, touch serves as an important mechanism of emotional release and communication. After reaching apparent psychological maturity we continue to need nonsexual sensual input through our skin.

* Touching: The Human Significance of the Skin (New York: Columbia University Press, 1971), p. 84.

Communication through the Skin

Throughout life we use the skin as a tension reliever. We finger our ears or stroke our chin when we think. We tug at our earlobes. We knead our foreheads and rub our closed eyes. We scratch our skin, pick our noses, wring our hands, and tap our fingers.

We use skin sensation to transmit both sexual and nonsexual messages. The extent to which we stimulate the skin of others in social contact is restricted by rules of society and etiquette, since sexual messages must generally be avoided in public. Still, men slap each other's backs or give firm two-handed handshakes, and athletes may pat each other on the buttocks as a gesture of reassurance or congratulation without fear of sexual interpretation. Women express sympathy and nonsexual affection by grasping hands and by embracing each other. The skin communicates our emotions to others even without touching. A blush graphically displays embarrassment, surprise, or pleasure. Facial pallor may express fear that is otherwise well concealed.

The skin is central to sexual arousal. Stimulation of the genital skin automatically alters blood flow in the underlying tissues, in both sexes. Nonerogenous zones are also highly sensitive to sexual messages, however. Holding hands, touching knees below the table, lightly stroking the back of the neck, gently twisting the hairs of the forearm — indeed, any contact — may communicate sexual desire and begin the cascade of physical and psychological preparations for intercourse.

The skin communicates with our environment and with other people at conscious and unconscious levels, for our protection and for our pleasure, from birth to death. It behooves us to know something about this tireless spokesman and interpreter.

16

4

Function and Structure of the Skin

FUNCTION OF THE SKIN

The skin is the covering of the body. It is a living organ that has assumed for higher animals the protective role performed by the cell walls of primitive single-celled organisms, such as bacteria. Mammals have an especially complex skin. Extensive hair growth prevents heat loss in cold climates and blocks the sun's rays in tropical areas. Claws, hooves, horns, nails, and scales afford protection against other animals and assist in locomotion and food-gathering. A large number and variety of skin glands secrete substances that lubricate the skin and hair or emit odors for protection, warning, or sexual attraction. Mammary glands, derived from the skin, nurture the young.

Men are "naked apes," distinguished from virtually all other mammals by their relative lack of fur. To compensate for this lack, human beings have developed a unique combination of features: a thick, well-developed outer layer of skin with a watertight coating, a widespread system of heat-sensitive sweat glands, an extensive layer of fatty tissue at the undersurface of the skin that serves as insulation and cushion, and a network of small blood vessels that constrict and expand to adjust the temperature both locally and throughout the body. This complex arrangement allows us to survive a wide range of temperatures and humidities.

Human beings are frequently exposed to heat and extreme cold, water, harsh chemicals, friction, and pressure. Skin must be tough and durable. It is also adaptable, thickening in areas of repeated trauma. Yet skin also permits easy mobility and allows underlying muscles and bones to perform complex movements. The skin must be strong enough to protect against direct assault, yet sensitive enough to pick up the many important but subtle messages about our environment that are also critical to our safety. Our covering must guard against a hostile world, yet be soft and delicate enough to allow our earliest, most meaningful, and most intimate forms of human communication.

Normal skin is a barrier, a first line of defense against germs, fluids, or chemicals entering the body. It also prevents loss of substances necessary for life and keeps the internal environment of the body relatively constant. The most fundamental barrier function of the skin is that of keeping water within the body. Water accounts for about 70 percent of body weight, yet we are surrounded by dry air. Our cells are bathed in salt water, an environment similar to that of the ocean, an expression of the sea as the origin of life. If water escapes freely from the body, we die. The skin's barrier properties keep the cells of internal tissues from drying out. Aside from sweat, which is carefully regulated by the skin, there is virtually no water loss. Conversely, we can also immerse ourselves in water for

18

hours without becoming waterlogged. Only the top layer of skin absorbs extra water.

Skin is more than a barrier. Its dry surface inhibits the growth of disease-causing microorganisms. The outer layer of skin is filled with small particles that absorb or reflect damaging radiation from the sun. The deeper layers of skin are tough and resilient, to modify deforming forces. Subcutaneous fat cushions the internal organs against physical trauma and insulates against heat exchange. The skin is also a sophisticated sensing device with a vast, complex network of nerves that provide information about our surroundings.

The skin is a complicated shell with protective physical and chemical characteristics that result from the constant activities of individual cells. Metabolic processes create the protective substances of the skin. The barrier is continually replaced, repaired, and maintained by living cells, which themselves are entirely replaced about once a month, every month of our lives.

The skin maintains a nearly constant thickness and is always just the right size for the body it covers.

STRUCTURE OF THE SKIN

The skin is the largest organ of the body. It accounts for about 15 percent of the total body weight and in an average adult is approximately two square yards in area. The thickness of the skin itself ranges from 1/50 inch (½ millimeter) over the eardrum or eyelids to well over ten times that thickness (up to ¼ inch) over the soles of the feet or the upper back. In most areas, a layer of fatty tissue adds to its thickness, while in some areas the skin lies directly on the underlying bone (as on the shin or hand) or cartilage (as on the outer ear).

The Epidermis

The epidermis is the outermost layer of skin. It is made up of ten to thirty closely packed cell layers but is only as thick as a sheet of paper. All the glands of the skin, as well as the hair and nails, are derived from the epidermis.

The cells that make up the epidermis are called *keratinocytes* because they produce *keratin*, the special protective protein of skin, which is also the major component of hair and nails, as well as fish scales, bird feathers, and the hooves, claws, and horns of other animals. *Basal cells* in the bottom layer of keratinocytes occasionally divide to create two new cells. One cell may remain in the basal layer while the other is pushed upward into the next layer of cells. This pattern creates a steady migration of cells to the skin surface. As each cell travels outward, it enlarges and flattens. The cells manufacture keratin, then lose their internal machinery, join firmly together, dehydrate, and eventually die. The final meshwork of flattened keratinocytes consists mostly of the protein keratin and is exceedingly resistant to chemical or physical breakdown. This outer covering is the *stratum corneum* or "horny layer."

The stratum corneum is dead. Its cells have no metabolic activity. It is the thinnest compartment of the skin in most body sites, often one-tenth the thickness of the living epidermal layer. If the epidermis is the thickness of a page in this book, the stratum corneum

20

is like print on the page. Still, there may be twenty or more layers of keratinocytes packed together like sheets of puff pastry. It is normally thick on the palms and soles and may thicken at any site as a response to repeated friction or pressure, forming a callus. In the stratum corneum, the keratinocytes are almost unrecognizable as individual cells, even under the microscope. Most of the barrier function of the skin resides in this thin outer layer of keratinocyte corpses.

Normally, it takes about two weeks for a cell to migrate from the basal layer to the stratum corneum and about two more weeks for that cell to be pushed through the stratum corneum to the outer surface of the skin. The top layer of the stratum corneum is constantly breaking up and sloughing off. We continuously shed dead cells at the same rate new cells are being made in the basal layer.

Melanocytes

Our pigment cells are at the base of the epidermis. Approximately every tenth cell in the basal layer is a *melanocyte*, a one-cell factory constantly producing small granules of a black-brown substance called *melanin*. These pigment granules give skin most of its color. The concentration of melanocytes varies about twofold from one body area to another, up to 1.5 million per square inch of skin surface, being greatest on the face and least on the trunk.

The purpose of melanocytes and their product, melanin, is not to provide differentiation among races through pigmentation nor to challenge the cosmetic industry to match the infinite number of human skin tones. Melanin protects us from the sun. Each pigment

21

granule can absorb ultraviolet light energy that would otherwise disrupt cells in the skin and damage the tissues below. Through the orderly process of evolution, people living in sunny tropical climates developed heavily pigmented skin, while those in northern climates developed fair complexions. In the latter case, protection from sunlight is not only unnecessary but harmful, since small amounts of ultraviolet light must enter the skin in order for vitamin D synthesis to occur. Ever since the Middle Ages, when man's ease of travel exceeded the rate of evolution, Caucasians living too near the equator have suffered from premature aging and skin cancer, while Africans and Asians in northern Europe developed rickets — at least until vitamin supplements were invented. (Chapter 12 discusses the more difficult and still growing problem of sun damage in fair-skinned people.) Tanning, the increased melanin pigmentation that occurs in most people after moderate sun exposure, is the body's attempt to protect individual cells and the skin as a whole from further sun damage.

All people have the same overall number of melanocytes, regardless of skin color. However, in a person with black skin, each melanocyte produces more melanin pigment and the individual pigment granules, or *melanosomes*, are much larger than those of a fair-skinned Caucasian. Orientals and others with brown skin tones produce intermediate amounts of melanin, packaged in intermediate-sized melanosomes.

Melanocytes are more like nerve cells than skin cells. Embryologically, they arise from the *neural crest*, the tissue that also forms the brain and peripheral nerves. During the third month of fetal development, they migrate from the region of the brain and spinal

Function and Structure of the Skin

cord to the skin. In the skin, melanocytes continue to resemble nerve cells. Each cell has many long arms or dendrites reaching out from its center to neighboring cells. Through its dendrites, one melanocyte maintains contact with approximately thirty-six epidermal cells and transfers to them pigment granules previously manufactured in the cell center. As the epidermal cells are pushed upward to the skin surface, they carry the granules with them. In this way, pigment is spread throughout the epidermis.

The baseline melanin production of each melanocyte is genetically determined, but the cells are quite sensitive to external influences and quick to increase or decrease this amount. The most common stimulus is sun exposure. Within minutes melanocytes shift already manufactured pigment granules from the center to the periphery of the cell. These intracellular pigment shifts cause a perceptible darkening of the skin tone that can last a day or more. A better-developed version of the same process of pigment shifts within melanocytes is responsible for color changes in chameleons. The melanocytes also begin to increase melanin production, so that about four days after the sun exposure the skin appears tanned. If no further sun exposure occurs, melanin production gradually returns to normal, and by two to four weeks the tan has disappeared. If sun exposure continues, melanin production remains above baseline.

Temporary dark spots frequently appear on the skin, especially in darkly pigmented people, after cuts, burns, rashes, or other minor skin injuries. This color change, like suntan, is a nonspecific response of the pigment cell to damage or insult experienced by the skin.

23

Epidermal Appendages

Early in fetal life small collections of the epidermal cells change in behavior and appearance. Complicated and poorly understood relationships between the dermis and the epidermis cause them to specialize. These cells make the appendages or "added structures" of the epidermis. Some of these specialized collections of epidermal cells give rise to the hair and nails. Other epidermal cells form the oil and sweat glands of the skin. These are not absolutely essential, but provide helpful "extras" — for example, without sweat glands, temperature control is severely impaired and in hot weather the body heat increases dangerously. A person born without sweat glands may have a temperature increase to 103°F during hot days. This is hardly surprising, considering that an adult may lose more than a half-gallon of sweat each hour in order to decrease body temperature through evaporation.

In the embryo, the appendages begin as buds of epidermal cells, protruding down into the dermis. As these cells multiply, the plug of cells becomes larger and extends down further into the dermis, which provides nutrients. Hair and sebaceous or oil glands arise together from the same clump of epidermal cells. As the cells multiply, the bud elongates, becomes hollow, and forms a tube. The epidermal cells at the base of the tube begin to make the keratin protein of hair, which differs slightly from the keratin in skin. Three bulges become apparent in the tubular column of cells. The uppermost bulge forms another column of cells that specialize to form an *apocrine* or vestigial scent gland and its duct. The middle bulge becomes a *sebaceous gland*, while the lower one becomes an attachment for a small *erector pili* muscle that can make body hairs stand

24

erect when stimulated by cold or strong emotion. *Eccrine* or sweat glands arise in a similar manner directly from the epidermis, without associated structures.

The hair, nails, and glands are epidermal in origin and character. The cells lining the ducts or walls of the appendages continue to look like keratinocytes and, indeed, these cells retain the ability to make stratum corneum under certain conditions. If the epidermis is removed by disease or trauma but the hair follicles in the dermis are left behind, the cells of the hair follicle walls migrate up to repopulate and resurface the injured area with normal keratinocytes.

The Dermis

The dermis is a thicker layer beneath the epidermis. It is tough and strong. A complex mixture of fluids and fibers creates a tissue with very high tensile strength that can resist compression but, at the same time, remains pliable and movable. Leather is animal dermis that has been modified by chemical treatments (tanning) which render it stable and resistant to decomposition or bacterial decay.

The dermis gives skin much of its substance or texture and provides structural support for the epidermis, for the skin glands and hair, and for blood vessels, nerves, and lymphatic channels. The dermis varies in thickness from about 1/20 to 3/20 inch (1½ to 4 millimeters) in different body areas. Whereas the epidermis is a continuous sheet of cells, the dermis is a semisolid gel of fibers and water, with only a few cells. Elongated, spindly cells called *fibroblasts* in the dermis produce the fibers and viscous materials. Throughout life, these cells constantly replace the substances that make

25

up the dermis and maintain its integrity. The dermis also contains scavenger cells that engulf and destroy foreign, unwelcome substances that find their way into the skin. At times of bacterial infection or other massive invasion, similar cells leave the bloodstream and join these cells in their protective role. The dead and dying bodies of these cells make up what we call pus.

The dermis envelops the whole body in a protective viscous gel that reduces environmental stress and strains on the internal organs. *Collagen* is a strong fibrous protein that makes up a large part of the dermis, 70 percent by dry weight. Individual molecules bind tightly together, side by side, forming collagen fibrils that then braid together as bundles that course through the skin. Collagen provides structure and is the major source of the skin's mechanical strength. This meshwork of fibers allows the skin to stretch and contract without damage. The laying down of new collagen, which is manufactured on location by the fibroblasts, is an important part of wound healing; scars represent excess collagen production. Normal collagen synthesis depends on vitamin C; vitamin C deficiency or scurvy causes poor healing and easily damaged skin.

The junction between epidermis and dermis is by no means flat. Per square inch the dermis has more than five hundred tiny fingerlike projections into the epidermis. These projections fit into corresponding sockets in the underside of the epidermis. Because of this arrangement, the interface between the two skin layers is many times larger than the surface area of the body. This large area of contact guarantees easy communication between the epidermis and dermis.

Nutrients and oxygen for the cells in the epidermis are brought by dermal capillaries and must diffuse out of the vessels, through the dermis and into the keratinocytes. Epidermal cell wastes and cell products intended to be resorbed and conserved by the body must make their way back to the dermal capillaries. Hair follicles, oil and sweat glands, and nail beds are surrounded by the dermis and also obtain nutrient supply by diffusion from the dermal vessels. The fluid that bathes the fibers and cells of the dermis also passes freely between the cells of the epidermis and stops only at the stratum corneum. An extremely thin barrier, the *basement membrane*, normally prevents cells and other large particles from traveling between the epidermis and dermis.

Subcutaneous Tissue

Beneath the dermis, fibrous proteins become loosely textured and, in most areas of the body, separated by collections of fat cells. This layer is called the *subcutaneous tissue*. In most body areas, it is much thicker than the dermis, but in some regions such as the eyelids, penis and scrotum, nipples, and shin it is absent. The thickness and fat content of the subcutaneous layer in various parts of the body are influenced by heredity, hormones, age, and eating habits. The different distribution of fatty tissue in males and females also constitutes one of the secondary sex characteristics.

Subcutaneous tissue is an insulator to conserve body heat. It is also an excellent shock absorber to reduce the effects of trauma on deeper structures. In the eye socket, fatty tissue acts as the perfect packing material to cushion the eyeball. Fat tissue is also a source of fuel. When adequate calories are not available from other sources, the fat cell provides needed energy.

27

5
Hair
and Nails

Hair and nails arise from the epidermis during fetal life and are fully formed at birth. Hair and nails are dead, but they are made by epidermal cells that are very much alive. Throughout life, their condition reflects the health of the skin and of the entire body.

Hairs begin to form in the third month of intrauterine life, first on the head and scalp, and eventually over the entire body surface except for the palms, soles, and lips. Clumps of keratinocytes in the fetal epidermis suddenly begin to divide more rapidly than their neighbors and the excess cells produced in this process grow downward into the dermis. Each clump of cells forms a hair follicle and a sebaceous gland, apparently intended, earlier in the evolutionary process, to lubricate the hair. The clump joins the small erector pili muscle, another vestigial structure that in man is not under voluntary control and can be used only to make the hairs become more erect ("gooseflesh"). At birth, the epidermis loses its ability to form new hair follicles, although the cells lining hair follicles can always revert to standard keratinocytes, migrate back to the surface, and rebuild missing areas of skin if necessary.

During gestation, the follicles produce *lanugo hair*, which is usually thin and silky and covers most of the body surface, somewhat resembling an animal's undercoat. Lanugo hair generally falls out just before birth but may persist for the first weeks of extrauterine life.

Hair growth is continuous in some animals such as poodles and Merino sheep. Each follicle produces one hair continuously from before birth until the animal's death. In most animals, however, including man, hair growth is cyclic. As a cycle begins, the entire hair follicle enlarges and grows farther downward into the dermis. Cells lining the inside of the follicle begin to multiply and the new cells are pushed together centrally to form the hair shaft, much as cells in the epidermis are pushed upward to form the stratum corneum. A hair grows in each follicle for a period called the *anagen phase*. Then growth stops and the follicle enters a resting period called the *telogen phase*. Between the growing and resting period is a brief *catagen phase* when the follicle shrinks to its pre-anagen size. Eventually the follicle again enlarges below the resting hair and begins to manufacture a new hair. The old hair is pushed out as the new hair begins to grow beneath it in the same follicle.

In many animals, the hair growth cycles are synchronized: all hairs grow at the same time and are then shed at the same time. In this way, Arctic hares and certain other animals grow a brown coat in summer, then replace it with a white coat in winter. In man, the hair cycles are asynchronous. At any point in time, some hairs are growing, others resting. The proportion of resting and growing hairs remains constant, so the scalp and other body areas are equally hairy year-round. Resting hairs are scattered evenly among grow-

29

Hair and Nails

ing ones, so that normal hair loss occurs continuously and inconspicuously, one hair here and another there, never a clump of hairs together.

On the normal adult scalp, about 85 percent of hairs are in the growing phase and 15 percent in the resting phase. The hairs that have stopped growing usually rest in place for several months before they are pushed up and out of the follicles when a new growth cycle begins within those follicles. We normally lose about seventy-five to one hundred scalp hairs per day through this continuous process. Growth phases for individual hairs vary from months to years on various parts of the body. Since all hairs grow at about the same rate, the duration of the growing phase determines how long a hair will be. A woman with long hair-growth cycles may sport waistlength tresses, while another person's hair may never reach below midback, no matter how long it is allowed to "grow." Scalp hairs, which remain in growth phase for up to six years, become very long, while eyelashes or hairs on limbs, which only grow for a few months, are much shorter.

During the growth phase, cells at the base of hair follicles reproduce approximately every twenty-four hours. Metabolic activity and cell multiplication rate in the hair follicle rank among the highest of any of the body tissues. An individual scalp hair grows about 1/80 inch or ⅓ millimeter each day, one inch each two to three months. Since there are about 100,000 scalp hairs, this growth produces about a hundred feet of solid protein thread each day, seven miles per year.

There are three ways in which hair growth expresses itself and by which it can be measured: growth cycle (length of the growth phase vs. length of the resting phase), rate of growth during the growth phase, and the diameter of each hair shaft produced. A change in any of these parameters in a large number of hairs leads to noticeable abnormalities.

A change in the hair cycle disturbs the regular pattern of growth. Hairs may prematurely stop growing and become resting hairs before reaching their usual length. A greater proportion of hairs than usual may enter the resting state. In cases of severe physical or emotional stress, all growing hairs may make this conversion and then all fall out together. As new hairs begin to grow in these follicles, the old hairs are all displaced at nearly the same time and thinning or near-balding may occur temporarily before the new hairs become obvious. This phenomenon probably accounts for the tales of hair falling out after a bad fright. It may also occur after pregnancy, severe illness, high fever, or the use of certain medications.

Environment and one's general state of health also change the rate of hair growth. Warm weather stimulates and cold climates reduce the growth of hair and nails, but these changes are not noticeable unless the environmental changes are extreme and prolonged. Starvation, certain anticancer drugs, and X rays may impair metabolism and reduce growth rate in the hair bulb so that the hair being made is narrower than usual. Although the hair bulb will re-expand and once again produce a hair of normal diameter when the inhibition is withdrawn, a segment of constriction remains in the hair. This narrow segment is pushed outward as hair growth continues below it. When the constriction reaches the skin surface, the hair may then break easily. For this reason, hair may seem unusually brittle or fragile for a time after a major illness.

Hair growth in many body areas is under hormonal control. Androgen, or testosterone, the male sex hormone, has the greatest influence in both sexes. Hair follicles in each part of the body have their own innate sensitivity to the hormone. Large amounts, made in the testicles after puberty, are necessary to stimulate beard growth, for example. In most men, the same hormone levels eventually cause at least some hair follicles on the scalp to shrink rather than grow and subsequently to produce only very fine short hairs, called *vellus* hairs. This conversion from large to small hairs is called "male pattern hair loss" (although in fact hairs persist), because the general appearance is that of a receding hairline or even complete baldness. Very small amounts of testosterone, made in the female ovaries and in the adrenal glands of both sexes, are sufficient to stimulate hair growth in the pubic area and under the arms.

Whether a hair is curly or straight depends upon its cross-sectional shape. Hair that is round, like a piece of spaghetti, remains straight as it grows. The more oval or ribbonlike a hair, the curlier it is. Intrinsically straight or curly hair can be altered, however. A beauty parlor permanent breaks chemical bonds within the hair shaft itself, then allows the bonds to reform in a different configuration after the hair has been molded on rollers. Chemical hair straighteners work by the same principle.

Hair color, like skin color, is due to pigment granules made in melanocytes and transferred to the surrounding keratinocytes. But there are some differences. Epidermal melanocytes can make only one pigment, melanin. It is black-brown. Skin color depends principally on the amount and location of this single pigment. Melanocytes in hair bulbs can make one of two compounds, melanin or a chemically similar red-yellow pigment called *phaeomelanin*. The former pig-

32

ment makes hair appear brown, black, or blond, depending on concentration; the latter makes hair red. Melanocytes in follicles must produce more pigment for growing hairs than must their counterparts in the slower growing skin. Hair follicles on the scalp, which have by far the longest growing phase, demand the greatest pigment production. Perhaps for this reason, they frequently cease functioning during middle age. One by one, new scalp hairs appear that are devoid of pigment. Eventually, the mixture of white and normally pigmented hairs is perceived as gray.

Nails are equivalent to the claws of lower animals. They begin to form in the third intrauterine month. A thickened disk of epidermal cells sinks down into the dermis near the tips of the fingers and toes, and the invaginated group of cells begins to make a special kind of keratin protein that becomes the nailplate. The process is similar to the formation of stratum corneum or hair shafts. Frequently dividing basal cells provide daughter cells that are pushed outward as they manufacture protein. The protein-containing cell corpses become the hard substance called nail.

The specialized group of epidermal cells that makes the nailplate is called the *nail matrix*. The white *lunula* or half-moon seen through the thumbnail of most people is the distal part of the matrix. The matrix of the other fingers is usually hidden by the skin that covers the base of the nail plate. The thin layer of protein and dead cells made by this skin fold grows over the base of the nail and is called the cuticle. Nail plate keratin is normally clear, and the pink color of blood vessels in the nail bed can be seen through it.

The nails grow continuously and would extend indefinitely if the free edge were not broken, worn away,

33

or deliberately cut. Nails are 1/30 to 1/50 inch thick and grow at a rate of about ⅛ inch each month. Nails of the right hand grow very slightly faster than corresponding nails of the left hand; middle fingernails grow faster than the rest; toenails grow only one-third to one-half as fast as fingernails. Like hair follicles, nail-forming tissue is very active metabolically and therefore very sensitive to physiologic alterations, such as serious illness or pregnancy.

Any skin disease that affects the epidermis can alter the nails and often does.

Hair and Nails

6
Life on
the Skin

The skin provides warmth, microscopic nooks and crannies that are hospitable to life, and nourishment for a large population of germs. Water is available from sweat and normal water loss through the epidermis. Amino acids, carbohydrates, and even some vitamins are available for food. Those organisms which can digest fats have additional food available from an oily material called *sebum* and epidermal cell fats.

The first bacteria to grow on a newborn's sterile skin come from the mother's vagina. Many more arrive in the first hours in the newborn nursery. Gradually, an elaborate ecology system is established. Various microorganisms transiently colonize the skin at the sites of contact, but because of special properties that vary greatly over different parts of the body, a characteristic flora eventually develops in each body site.

Throughout your life, these microorganisms eat, multiply, compete with each other for space, die, and sometimes spread to other people. Mites live, mate, and have their offspring in the hair follicles of your eyelashes and face. Yeasts prefer the moist areas of your body. Fungi may quietly digest the dead stratum corneum on your feet. Viruses that attack bacteria are plentiful on the surface of the skin.

Bacteria dominate the society of microorganisms on normal human skin. Harmless species of staphylococci and diphtheroids are major inhabitants of almost all regions of the skin. In fact, their presence seems to exert a restraining force on colonization from other, perhaps more dangerous, organisms to which the skin is constantly exposed. Some bacteria even produce antibiotics that kill off competing species.

The absolute number of bacteria and the ranking of species vary from one body region to another. The trunk is a desert compared with the tropical rain forest of the armpits. The scalp, a shady protected area, harbors many bacteria. The moist, warm genital area welcomes bacteria from the anus and vagina. The proportion changes, but the same few kinds of bacteria make up the residents of most areas. The populations are relatively stable, but the hands are constantly smearing colonies of bacteria from place to place. Organisms settle on the skin from the air. Minute scales that fall off the body become airborne, providing a flying carpet to carry the bacteria to other people.

Some bacteria reside on the uppermost stratum corneum, but the most superficial cells of the stratum corneum provide an inhospitable, dry atmosphere. Bacterial colonies prefer more protected, moist creases, the deep furrows of the skin markings, and the folds in the skin. An exception is the face with its microscopic layer of sebum, which provides a pleasant, greasy covering. The sebaceous follicles of the face are gaping holes filled with nutritious sebum for bacteria adapted to the eating of oils.

36   Even though free food, water, and housing are pro-

vided, bacteria do not overwhelm the skin. The depth of bacterial penetration is limited by the barrier layer, the stratum corneum. The skin is constantly being shed, hair and nails grow outward, the sebum is pushed out onto the surface. New sterile skin cells push up from below. The skin's acid pH and the presence of fatty acids discourage the growth of some organisms, but the protective importance of these factors has probably been overemphasized in the past. The enzymes and metabolic products provided by normal resident flora discourage the growth of other unfamiliar, potentially disease-causing bacteria. Antibodies circulating in the bloodstream and other immunologic reactions may also aid in the defense of the skin against certain organisms.

Scrubbing the hands removes some surface bacteria, but colonies remain in the microscopic creases of the skin. Bacterial counts on the skin may actually increase after showering or bathing, since increased skin temperature, dilatation of pores, and vigorous toweling may open the deep bacterial reservoirs and spread bacteria over the skin. Those who dislike washing must not leap to conclusions, however: the process is not dangerous.

The bacteria usually found on normal skin are there because they are best adapted to the habitat provided by the skin, and because they have proven harmless over countless generations.

7

Care of
Normal Skin—
Soaps and Cosmetics

The purpose of skin care for most people is to prevent disease, to sustain health. In the case of this most visible organ of our bodies, we are also concerned with aesthetics, with maintaining and enhancing an image of youth and vigor and beauty. And proper skin care is surprisingly easy. Why is it so rarely practiced, despite this widespread interest and concern?

In many ways it is like good eating habits. We all know how to remain slender and healthy. Nutrition charts and calorie guides are readily available, and eating well is usually a matter of common sense. The correct foods are on the grocer's shelf. Still, we choose to overeat much of the time, to overindulge in "empty calories" or alcoholic beverages, which not only lack food values but are potentially dangerous to our mental and physical health. To compensate for these excesses, we periodically diet or even stop eating altogether. Many people have frequent fluctuations of up to 20 percent of their body weight as a result of such off-again, on-again eating habits. No one can deceive himself into thinking that this is better than eating a balanced diet every day. We also try to buy our way out. Many an otherwise thrifty housewife buys expensive dietetic jams to atone for those extra slices of toast. Because we are undisciplined, we behave in this way in spite of our knowledge of and genuine commitment to a healthy diet.

We care for our skin in the same way, for the same reasons. It is now well-known that chronic sun exposure is the leading cause of "premature aging" changes in skin. We know that the best care we can give our skin is to protect it over the years from adverse environmental factors—from excessive sun, cold, wind, dryness and harsh chemicals. Such advice not only is forthcoming from numerous authorities but is plain common sense. Yet the most appearance-conscious young woman spends her summers at the beach in a bikini, her winters on the ski slopes without a face mask or sunscreen, and never wears rubber gloves to do housework. Instead of taking steps to prevent damage to her skin, she has a monthly facial or buys an expensive moisturizing cream. While at the beach, she uses an ultrachic but usually ineffective lotion or cream to prevent sunburn. Her hands are ignored until a rash or painful cracks appear, then they receive the best care money can buy—until the symptoms end. Men and women are equally guilty of such behavior.

Every dermatologist wishes there were a cream or pill to reverse skin damage and aging. Such a medicine does not exist. Every sunburn, every windburn causes slight but irreversible changes in the skin that accumulate over the years and eventually become obvious as wrinkling, sagging, blotchy pigmentation, and even skin cancer. Although many products provide temporary improvement in appearance and comfort, they are a poor substitute for proper skin care and the prevention of damage.

Care of Normal Skin—Soaps and Cosmetics

If you are to retain youthful and healthy skin, you must make a lifelong, everyday commitment to rational skin care. It's not that difficult. Much easier, in fact, than eating properly!

WASHING: HOW OFTEN?
WHAT TYPE OF CLEANSER?

Washing, for many persons, serves more than its original function of removing dirt and has become a symbol, a ritual. For many people, the daily bath may be the only moment of relaxation and self-indulgence in a busy day; the morning shower may be as necessary as a cup of coffee for fully waking up. For the acne-prone adolescent, scrubbing the face six times a day may even be a veiled attempt at self-destruction. We now know that washing is almost unnecessary for healthy skin, except occasionally to remove bacteria and fungi that might otherwise initiate infection. It is a societal dictate. Therefore, the frequency and vigor of washing should be adjusted to the amount of dirt, sweat, and other body secretions that accumulate to the point of being noticed. In general, washing once a day is ample. Washing the entire skin only every two or three days may be quite adequate for small children or older adults.

In "polite society," it is rare to find a person who bathes too little, but many people wash too frequently. Certain bacteria and microorganisms form a normal and probably necessary part of the microenvironment of the skin. Likewise, certain materials that we may think of as dirt or soil are natural end products of the

40

"skin machine," a sign of healthy skin; in no way do they inhibit the efficient functioning of our protective covering, as a speck of dust may impair the machinery of a watch or a turntable. Totally dust-free, antiseptic, shiny cleanliness may be the standard for precision instruments but not for skin.

There are seven principal types of soil, including these natural by-products of the "skin machine," as well as "pollutants" from the environment and materials purposely applied to the skin. These are (1) dead skin cells, (2) excess natural oils, (3) salts and other components of sweat, (4) microorganisms such as bacteria and fungi, (5) airborne dust and pollens, (6) miscellaneous chemicals and other matter picked up in a job or hobby, and (7) cosmetics, ointments, lotions, and creams.

Most soils probably are harmless, and the main reason for their removal is aesthetic, but some soils (strong acids, for example) will seriously injure the skin if they are not promptly removed. Most cosmetics will do no harm, especially if the normal practice of cleaning the skin between applications is followed.

In terms of skin cleansing, we can divide skin soils into three groups: water-soluble, oil-soluble, and insoluble. The latter two are, of course, more difficult to remove than the first. Water not only will remove water-soluble soils, it will "float off" some insoluble soils if they are not held fast to the skin by natural oils or other oily soils.

The oldest and most commonly used cleanser is soap. Technically, soap is a sodium or potassium salt of fatty acids; it is a type of surfactant. Used with warm water, it will satisfactorily remove nearly all types of soil from normal skin. While it doesn't dissolve oils, it disperses or emulsifies them in very fine droplets,

41

which are suspended in the soapy water. The air bubbles in lather possibly help by lifting the soils farther off the skin, so that they can be more easily rinsed away.

The tremendous varieties of cleansing products available in the grocery store or pharmacy differ from one another chiefly by reason of their additives: perfumes, artificial coloring, moisturizers, and antibacterial agents. Soaps for acne patients also usually contain agents to make them abrasive and drying; they are discussed in Chapter 23. Here we will consider only soaps intended for normal or "sensitive," nearly normal skin.

The question of which soap is probably less important than the question, "How often?" Virtually all skin can tolerate occasional exposure to any commercially available soap without becoming irritated. On the other hand, very frequent use of even the mildest soap may produce undesirable changes. For most people, the choice of soap can safely be based on such factors as cost, fragrance, and "image." As long as the skin is clean, comfortable, and normal in appearance, there is no need for concern. Moreover, there are few scientific data on which to base a choice. Soaps are not under regulation by the Food and Drug Administration and hence manufacturers are not required to prove their efficacy or to substantiate advertising claims of "mildness," a vague concept in any case.

Superfatted soaps, which are simply regular soaps with a little extra fat in them, are said to make the skin smoother by depositing fat on it. If, in fact, they do deposit oil on the skin — and there is no convincing evidence that they do — they could hardly cleanse it thoroughly, since one of the objectives of using soap is to remove oil. Some people believe that superfatted soaps are less drying than regular soaps. If this were

42

true, it would probably be at the expense of cleansing effectiveness. One caveat: people with acne or with a tendency for acne (and this includes most of us under the age of thirty-five) should avoid using these "creamy" or "moisturizing" soaps on their faces, upper backs, and chests, since such products may encourage acne lesions (Chapter 23).

Some of the newer synthetic detergents appear to be more effective cleansers than soap. In hard water they also are pleasanter to use than soap, because they do not form a precipitate. (It is the precipitate that causes bathtub ring and has an unpleasant feel on the skin.) Most of the new detergents remove accidentally acquired oily soils, applied oils, and natural oils more easily than soaps do. They may be too efficient in this respect for people with skin that is deficient or even normal in production of natural oils. Among the bar-form detergents now available are Dove®, Vel®, and Zest®; if the use of ordinary toilet soap appears objectionable for any reason, bar detergents are worth trying.

Waterless, solvent-type skin cleansers, which are rubbed on and wiped off, are used in many work places. Waterless cleansers are good oil solvents and dispersing agents and do an efficient job of cleaning badly soiled skin. However, the organic solvents they contain irritate some skins.

The regular use of antiseptic soaps such as Dial® or Lifebuoy®, which reduce bacterial growth by depositing an antiseptic on the skin, appears to diminish but not eliminate body odor in most people. Most skin secretions, including sweat, are odorless at first and develop an odor only after bacterial decomposition. Routine washing with regular soap will remove some of the bacteria responsible and some of the odorous

43

Care of Normal Skin—Soaps and Cosmetics

products, but regular soaps are not quite as effective as the antiseptic soaps. There is no convincing evidence that such soaps can prevent skin infections or alleviate acne, which results in part from the presence of bacteria.

It bears repeating that if your skin feels dry, you should wash less often, wash more gently, and wash less thoroughly. Hands are especially at risk, since many occupations and avocations seem to require frequent hand-washing. Anyone who must wash more than three or four times a day should use a moisturizer such as petrolatum immediately after washing. This is true for backyard gardeners, health professionals, and industrial workers. It is especially important if certain solvents or harsh detergents are used. Or you can try alternating soap and water with a cleansing cream or a synthetic detergent, or after washing apply a simple oily skin lotion or an aqueous solution of glycerin (glycerin and rose water), which may help hold more water in the outer layer of skin.

A few people have more severe reactions from the use of soap, but even in the rare cases where this represents a true allergy, the cause is more likely to be a dye, perfume, or antiseptic in the soap than the soap itself. The specially formulated "mild" soaps, such as Neutrogena®, Lowila®, Keri®, and Dove® are preferred by many people who complain of "sensitive skin," though there is no proof that they are less irritating than standard brands.

We know far too little about the effect of any soap on the skin to make firm recommendations. A trial-and-error approach, guided by advertising claims, is the best you can do. But whichever soap you choose, use it sparingly.

44

WHAT ELSE SHOULD YOU USE ON YOUR SKIN?

Many products, promoted for regular use, are intended in the long run to protect or improve the skin. Moisturizers, facial packs, vitamin E creams, and astringents are but a few examples.

In general, these substances are harmless. Some may produce mild irritant reactions and, of course, any of them may in rare cases cause allergic contact dermatitis (Chapter 28). None of them is necessary. None has been shown to have any long-term effect on the skin, good or bad.

Cold creams, cleansing creams, washing creams, moisturizing creams, and night creams are all variations on a theme. All contain the same basic ingredients — oil, wax, and water — in different proportions. The oil may be animal, vegetable, or mineral in origin; beeswax or any of several synthetic waxes are used. Today almost all products of this type also contain perfume and preservatives. Many contain, in addition, one or more "special" ingredients such as hormones, vitamins, collagen, protein, algae, aloe, or fruit extracts. *None of these additives has been shown to have a beneficial effect on skin.* Many do not even penetrate through the skin barrier. It is very difficult to accept the fact that advertising in the media is so flagrantly misleading or that manufacturing companies are allowed to perpetrate such a hoax on the public. We want to believe the ads. Nevertheless, creams do *not* rejuvenate or beautify skin, no matter how expensive, how pleasant to apply, or how attractively advertised. They do "soften" the skin temporarily by coating the normally somewhat irregular surface with an oil film and by re-

45

tarding water loss. Like soaps, creams of this type also emulsify oil and dirt particles on the skin surface. However, for routine cleansing, soap and water are more effective than creams, which are never completely removed when the skin is wiped with a cloth or tissue. "Special ingredients" add nothing to the emollient or cleansing properties of such creams.

Astringents and skin fresheners contain alcohol in combination with other ingredients. They make the skin feel cool and "tight" as the alcohol evaporates. Overuse can dry skin; no amount of these products can "shrink pores" or otherwise alter the structure of the skin. The same is true of facial packs, whether made from mud or any of the hundreds of exotic bases. These compounds draw water from the skin as they dry, causing a pleasant "tight" or tingling sensation. If truly irritating substances are added to the facial pack, the skin swells slightly, making the face appear less wrinkled and pores less prominent until the irritation subsides, usually after several hours. A bad sunburn has the same effect.

The decision to use such substances should be based on the short-term benefits you derive. Moisturizing or emollient creams do indeed retard water loss from the skin surface. If you have dry skin, applying such a cream after your bath when the skin is hydrated will make it look and feel smoother for many hours. However, faithful use of an emollient will not prevent your skin from becoming dry in the future, if it is so destined either by heredity or by abuse, such as excessive sunbathing.

Two imported customs for bathing may be of special benefit to the skin: the Japanese bath and the French bidet. The Japanese bath is intended not for cleansing but for its relaxing and moisturizing effects. After

46

showering or bathing with soap and rinsing thoroughly, the bather sits in a deep tub, made traditionally of an aromatic wood, filled only with clean, hot water. For those with dry skin, the procedure can be modified by adding bath oil (for example, Alpha-Keri®) to the water and by applying a moisturizing cream to the entire skin surface immediately after toweling dry, to trap water in the skin.

The bidet is a basin designed to clean the anogenital area. It is standard bathroom equipment in French and many other European and South American homes but has never gained popularity in the United States. It is curious that Americans, with their almost compulsive cleanliness and fastidious attention to underarms and mouth, often neglect that area which is most difficult to clean. Regular use of a bidet after bowel movements or urination is especially helpful for people with pruritus ani or pruritus vulvae (Chapter 20), irritations of the anogenital region that are aggravated by poor hygiene. Also, simple cleansing of the anogenital area with warm water in a bidet before and after intercourse is easier and more effective than showering, bathing, or applying deodorant sprays.

DEODORANTS AND ANTIPERSPIRANTS

Most people use at least one deodorant or antiperspirant product daily to control perspiration and body odor. There are products specially formulated for underarms, for genital regions, and for the feet.

Axillary (underarm) sweat stains clothing. Profuse sweating dampens palms and soles and predisposes to

47

athlete's foot infection. However, it is the action of bacteria on secretions from the skin's glands, not the secretions themselves, that causes body odor. There can be little doubt that regular, effective bathing is the primary means of controlling this bacterial growth on the skin.

These bacteria, known as resident bacteria, are commonly found on everyone's skin and are most active in warm, moist surroundings. Three types of glands in the skin produce secretions on which bacteria can work.

Eccrine sweat glands are relatively unimportant in odor formation because eccrine sweat has only trace amounts of organic material on which bacteria can act. These glands primarily help to control body temperature by providing the surface of the skin with water for evaporative cooling. They are usually active only during exercise or nervous tension or when the temperature is high. But in certain areas of the body, such as the palms and soles and underarms, they produce perspiration at lower temperatures and may become particularly active as a result of emotional stress. In some persons, certain foods, especially spices, activate the eccrine sweat glands.

Apocrine sweat glands, in contrast, produce perspiration that is rich in organic material for bacterial action. Also, these glands are concentrated in the axillae, around the nipples, and in the genital area, ideal sites for bacterial growth since moisture cannot readily evaporate there. Apocrine glands become active only after puberty and remain active as long as the sexual glands are active. Apocrine sweat glands are stimulated by fear, pain, and sexual excitement, but not by heat.

Care of Normal Skin—Soaps and Cosmetics

The third type, the sebaceous glands, lubricate the skin with the oily sebum. They play a relatively minor role in body odor in persons who bathe regularly.

Dermatologists generally believe that the products excreted by all three types of glands are odorless, or nearly so, at the time of secretion. Odors become manifest very suddenly, however, during emotional stress. Since it is doubtful that this is the result only of immediate bacterial activity, a theory has been suggested to explain the phenomenon: substances within the ducts of the glands that have already decomposed may be spread over the surface of the skin by the increased gland activity. Evaporation from the larger area thus covered could quickly make the presence of these products apparent.

In any event, there are two methods to prevent body odor: impede bacterial action and reduce the secretion of perspiration. Deodorant soaps and deodorants are intended to accomplish the former; antiperspirants may do both. Indeed, a few deodorants depend mainly on odor substitution, their perfume temporarily masking a disagreeable odor with a more pleasant one. A shopper generally can tell which type of product he or she is buying by examining the label. The active ingredients of antiperspirants must be listed because these products affect a body function (sweating) and are therefore considered drugs under the federal Food, Drug and Cosmetic Act. The active ingredients of a deodorant, which is considered a cosmetic under federal law, may or may not be listed. Thus, any body-odor preventive that does not show a list of ingredients may be assumed to be a simple deodorant.

One probably gets longer-lasting protection against bacteria in the underarm area with a deodorant con-

Care of Normal Skin—Soaps and Cosmetics

taining an antiseptic than with soaps containing an antiseptic, because more of the deodorant chemical remains on the skin. The simple application of a deodorant cannot, however, remove bacteria. Such an application is not a substitute for cleansing and should follow adequate bathing.

A few years ago, chlorophyllins were widely promoted as the answer to all odor problems — in tablets, mouth washes, lozenges, toothpastes, skin preparations, dog foods, and were even impregnated into clothing. It is now clear that chlorophyllins have no regular or lasting effect on either body or mouth odor.

Recently, it has been suggested that neomycin and other antibiotics in skin preparations could control underarm odor by inhibiting bacterial growth. Although effective, such preparations could induce allergic reactions in some individuals, encourage the development of strains of microorganisms resistant to the antibiotics, and promote the development of yeast infections. If such products should be marketed, consumers would do well to think twice before using them.

Many antiperspirants contain some type of aluminum salt. Like the antiseptics used in deodorants, these salts retard bacterial multiplication. In addition, they can reduce the amount of sweat that reaches the skin surface. Their effectiveness seems to vary from person to person and from time to time, so it is wise to buy the smallest available container of a new brand until you know that it works for you.

Antiperspirants in current use are relatively inefficient in the control of profuse sweating or for perspiration of the palms and soles, which some people find much more troublesome than underarm perspiration. At best the amount of sweat can be reduced by half.

50

Care of Normal Skin—Soaps and Cosmetics

All deodorants and antiperspirants do what their advertisers claim: they temporarily reduce sweating and/or body odor. Prescription agents and, rarely, special procedures available from a dermatologist or other physician may help people for whom the usual products have failed.

PRODUCTS FOR HAIR

Hair can be altered to a far greater degree than can skin. It can be curled or straightened, bleached or dyed. Products that promise to change the appearance of hair usually do, and safely, when used according to instructions. The intended misconceptions among consumers arise, as in the case of skin care products, when manufacturers capitalize on the desire to have hair that not only *looks* better for the moment but *is* better. There are innumerable products for washing and conditioning hair. Like skin creams, these products frequently contain "special ingredients." However, the hope that eggs, gelatin, other types of protein, beer, herbs, or fruit juices can improve hair is even less realistic than the claims for skin creams. Hair is dead. Nothing can alter its chemical composition or its thickness. Protein shampoos or rinses do not improve the hair's nutritional status. Because these products are inherently sticky, they may leave a thin coating on the hairs, giving the appearance of body, and may glue together fragments of split ends. These effects are real, but only temporary and superficial, like the benefits of skin creams.

51

CONCLUSIONS

Rational skin care requires self-confidence in the face of aggressive advertising, a bit of experimentation to find those products best suited to individual needs, and, above all, a willingness to accept the fact of damaged or imperfect skin, if it exists. Preventing unnecessary injury is the greatest service you can do your skin, and it is one too often forgotten.

8

Variations of Normal Skin—Changes throughout Life

The skin of the newborn usually becomes a red-blue during delivery but appears increasingly pink to red over the next several hours. This redness normally fades over two to three days and is often followed by a fine scaling. This generalized scaling is a response to mild irritation during birth and may be impressive in some infants, especially on hands and feet. Such scaling is a normal event and not a cause for concern.

Because muscle tone of the small blood vessels in the skin is not fully functional at birth, blood distribution in the infant's skin may appear abnormal. Blood tends to pool in the dependent portions of the body, and skin may have poor or intermittent circulation. Blotchy red, white, or purplish areas may appear after a baby cries or if the baby's room temperature is low. A harmless but striking color change may occur when an infant is lying on its side. The half of its body that is uppermost may suddenly become pale, while the lower half flushes red, exactly to the midline. The colors of the two sides reverse when the child is turned to the opposite side. Localized swelling of the skin may also occur. These changes are intermittent, reversible, and rarely of any significance.

Colonization of the skin by bacteria begins immediately after birth. Infants obtain bacteria first from the vaginas of their mothers, then from all who handle them, as well as from nursery objects and airborne particles. Within a few weeks the organisms normally present on adult skin exist on the infant's skin. The establishment of the normal, harmless bacteria on the skin is important because their presence helps prevent invasion by disease-producing organisms.

At birth, the skin is frequently covered with a greasy or cheesy film called the *vernix caseosa*. This film is largely composed of products from the infant's sebaceous glands mixed with sloughed skin and dried amniotic fluid. The vernix usually washes or wears off in a few days.

A baby's skin is thin and has a poorly developed barrier layer. Heat, cold, sunlight, and chemicals pass through it easily. Hot water or beverages spilled on a small child may cause third-degree burns, whereas the same accident would cause only brief discomfort for an adult. Moderate sun exposure may lead to blistering. Use of diapers previously stored in mothballs may result in sufficient absorption of the chemical naphthalene to produce severe anemia. Since many substances can cause allergies or disease after penetrating the skin, chemicals or medications should never touch a baby's delicate skin without a doctor's prior approval.

The epidermal appendages may not be fully developed at birth. Tiny white cysts called *milia* commonly appear scattered over the face. These represent partially developed, faulty, or plugged hair follicles. Milia

54

may form because maternal hormones stimulate secretion of oil into follicles that are not yet mature and fully open.

The amount of scalp hair present at birth is quite variable. Frequently only fine vellus hairs, like those on an adult's "hairless" skin, are present and the baby appears bald; but most infants have some terminal (easily visible) hairs on their scalps. Most scalp hairs are in the resting phase at birth. These resting hairs are dislodged as new hairs begin to grow in the follicles and so fall out over the ensuing weeks, making the child appear even balder. Rubbing of the baby's head on the crib often accelerates the normal shedding at the back or side of the scalp. It may take as long as six to twelve months before the asynchronized postnatal growth cycles become established to provide a constant number of scalp hairs at all times.

Maternal or placental hormones also influence the sex organs of the fetus. The newborn may have swollen, slightly enlarged sex organs or a well-developed vaginal lining with a white discharge. The breast tissue of both male and female infants may be engorged and may secrete small amounts of milk. These changes are all reversed within several weeks as the maternal sex hormones that entered through the placenta are metabolized by the infant's body. They do not affect the later normal development of the sex organs at puberty. Because sebaceous glands are also sensitive to maternal hormones, the infant's glands are transiently stimulated to develop and function like those of a teenager. For this reason, many babies have acne for the first several months of life. After a few months, sebaceous glands become quiescent until stimulated by hormones at adolescence.

Eccrine sweat glands may not function for several

55

days after birth, and even then they often cannot deliver large quantities of sweat. The immature sweat ducts may retain sweat within the skin and subsequently cause inflammation. Tiny red bumps called *miliaria* — prickly heat — occur at the site of such occluded glands. Whenever the body or environmental temperature rises and sweat glands begin to function, prickly heat reappears. Such lesions, once formed, may last for several days.

Three types of skin lesions occur so often in babies that they may be considered normal. Tiny pimples on a red base scattered on the face and trunk of newborns are signs of a condition called *erythema toxicum neonatorum*, but it is not at all toxic or infectious. The spots disappear without therapy in a few days or weeks.

Infants are usually plump with many skin folds. Moisture and friction cause an irritation and redness of the opposing surfaces of skin folds called *intertrigo*. If room temperature and humidity are high, babies are more likely to develop intertrigo. Invasion by yeast or bacteria may require treatment by a physician. In the absence of any complicating factors, however, the condition usually lasts only a few days or weeks. Mild cases can be cured by dressing the baby in looser, cooler clothing and by avoiding use of greasy ointment in body creases.

Diaper rash (*napkin dermatitis*) is an inflammatory reaction in areas normally covered by diapers. It occurs at some time in almost all infants but is also seen in older children and adults who have lost control over bladder function. The lower abdomen, buttocks, genital region, and upper thighs appear angry red. Scattered small pimples, bumps, or raw areas may be superimposed on the redness. The apex of the body creases may be less involved than the surrounding

56

skin, because the urine and feces in soiled diapers often do not reach these areas.

Diaper rash involves a combination of factors. Prolonged contact with urine damages the skin barrier. Rubber pants and diapers with outer plastic lining prevent evaporation and increase the damage. Bacteria are always present in feces and break down chemical wastes in the urine, causing more irritation. Prickly heat, discussed above, may add to the disorder. Soaps or chemicals left in the diaper because of poor laundering or to retard bacterial growth may further complicate the problem. Once irritation is present and the protective stratum corneum is damaged, the skin is far more susceptible and the cycle continues. Finally, certain bacteria or yeast may take advantage of the moisture and of the abundant food supply in feces to cause superinfection.

Diaper rash is best treated by thorough cleansing during each diaper change. Often all that is needed to cure diaper rash is to discontinue use of rubber or plastic pants, make frequent diaper changes (every hour when awake), allow air drying of the skin, and cleanse properly. In warm weather, the baby should be without a diaper as much as possible. Sometimes it helps to spread several diapers over the crib mattress during naps or at night so the baby does not have to sleep encased in a wet diaper. If a diaper is essential, use two cloth ones alone instead of one diaper covered by plastic pants. Disposable diapers are a wonderful convenience but should be avoided if possible in babies with severe or recurrent diaper rash. The skin appears clean after removal of a urine-soaked diaper, but, of course, it is not. The skin should not simply be wiped with a dry area of the diaper or a cloth, but rather washed with mild soap and thoroughly rinsed.

57

Towelettes that contain alcohol or perfume are very painful for injured skin. Quaternary ammonium compounds to kill bacteria may be used for laundering diapers at home, and commercial laundries now routinely use such rinses. For severe diaper rash, zinc oxide ointment, petrolatum, Vaseline®, or Desitin® ointment, which seems especially soothing and effective, should be applied during each diaper change. If this is not successful after a few days, a doctor may prescribe a steroid cream after checking the skin for infection.

CHILDHOOD

This is the golden age for skin. The blotches and rashes of infancy have disappeared; wear and tear are not yet visible. The sebaceous glands — the future site of acne lesions and source of numerous adult skin problems — barely function. Hair is present in all the socially correct places and absent in all the wrong ones. Nicks and cuts heal quickly with minimal scarring. There is no body odor. A brief and wonderful time.

ADOLESCENCE

Adolescence is a difficult period for most people, emotionally, socially, physically. The skin reflects the major changes that must occur in order for a child to become an adult.

58

At puberty, the gonads begin to secrete hormones that cause the genitalia to mature. In a boy, the male hormone androgen (testosterone) causes the penis and scrotum to enlarge to many times the preadolescent size. In a girl, the female hormone estrogen causes fat to deposit in the mons pubis and the labia majora. The vaginal lining thickens and changes its metabolism, becoming more resistant to mechanical trauma and infection. These and certain internal changes such as the growth of the testes or ovaries are the major sexual changes of adolescence. Other pubertal changes, the secondary ones, account for most of the difference in appearance between adult men and women. Many of these involve the skin.

In boys, testosterone causes the growth of large terminal hairs over the pubis upward along the midline of the lower abdomen, often to the navel. Testosterone also causes prominent hair growth on the face and chest, under the arms, and less often on other regions such as the back, arms, and legs. Male hormone affects the skin itself, causing it to increase in thickness over the entire body.

In girls, female hormones cause development of breast tissue and the deposit of fat throughout the breast. Estrogens cause or permit deposit of increased quantities of fat throughout the subcutaneous tissue, especially in the buttocks and thighs. The specific gravity or density of the female body is lower than that of the male body, because her body contains relatively less muscle, which is heavy, and more fat, which is light. For this reason, women float more easily in water than men do.

Testosterone is made by the adrenal glands of both sexes and by the female ovaries, as well as by the male

59

testes. The amount of this hormone in women is very low compared with that in men, but it is enough to cause prominent hair growth in the pubic region and under the arms. Indeed, hair growth in these areas usually begins before menarche (onset of menstruation), at the same time as early breast development. Women, like men, can grow hair in the beard area and on the chest, but only under the stimulation of supplemental testosterone, since the normal female hormone level allows only an occasional stray hair in these areas.

In both sexes, testosterone causes the glands in the skin to mature. Sebaceous glands enlarge and begin to produce oil. Acne appears (Chapter 23). Apocrine sweat glands under the arms and around the genitalia become active, resulting in body odor. Sweating from eccrine glands increases markedly in response to exercise or emotional stress. For the first time, good hygiene requires use of deodorants in addition to regular bathing. Sexual maturity invites sexual activity and the risk of venereal disease (Chapter 36).

Adolescence is a time of identity crisis, sexual awakening, increasingly difficult school work, and a first hard look at individual responsibility. These emotional stresses are often manifested in the skin. Conditions like eczema (Chapter 26) and psoriasis (Chapter 24), which have emotional aspects, may flare or appear for the first time. Small birthmarks or minor abnormalities of the skin may become major deformities in the mind of the adolescent.

Some adolescent skin characteristics such as acne tend to be left behind when the individual reaches adulthood. Most of the changes persist, but never again are they the source of such anxiety and fascination as they are at puberty.

60

ADULTHOOD

If we define adulthood for the skin as that time between adolescence and old age, it is a variable period indeed. Normal, stable function and appearance may last for as few as five years or as many as forty. The less sun-damaged the skin, the more retarded the changes that signal the end of this period. The very gradual, insidious deteriorations that begin in adolescence or early adulthood are discussed below in the section on old age, the period when they are most evident.

PREGNANCY

Virtually every part of a woman's body is affected by pregnancy. The skin is no exception. First, the skin must stretch over the pregnant uterus. Sometimes it stretches so rapidly and so far that the dermis develops small cracks called *striae* or "stretch marks," but often the skin accomplishes this amazing feat without the least damage.

Pigmentation is altered in certain body areas. The nipples darken and in many women a vertical brown line, the *linea nigra*, appears in the middle of the lower abdomen and slowly lengthens toward the navel as the uterus enlarges. *Melasma*, also called the mask of pregnancy, appears as spotty brown pigmentation on the cheeks and forehead and around the eyes. It is especially prominent in people of Mediterranean ancestry and in those who have had generous sun exposure. Indeed, the only way to erase the mask during pregnancy is by completely avoiding sun exposure to the face. An opaque sunscreen, such as A-Fil® or Reflecta®, or pancake-type makeup must be worn at all times. A nonprescription bleaching cream, such as Eldoquin®, Artra®, or Esoterica®, may also be applied morning and evening to the dark areas. Except for the temporary cosmetic liability, melasma is harmless and may be ignored.

Blood vessels as well as pigment cells are stimulated by the hormones of pregnancy. *Spider angiomas* are proliferations of small arteries that grow up toward the skin surface and look like small spiders or pinwheels. Most women develop at least a few and some women, hundreds. Veins in the legs often become prominent and tortuous, especially in the last trimester. Varicose veins may be, in part, a response to hormone changes but are due mainly to increased pressure inside the veins, which are compressed in the pelvis by the pregnant uterus.

Hair and nails usually grow faster than normal. The hair may seem unusually thick and lustrous.

The whole body is slightly warmer than usual during pregnancy, and this is reflected in the skin. Women perspire more readily; their hands and feet feel warmer. Yeast infections of the skin and vagina are more likely to occur during pregnancy, affecting about one woman in ten, in part because the skin folds are warmer and more moist.

Pregnancy often affects the course of chronic skin diseases such as acne, eczema, and psoriasis. The conditions may worsen, but usually they improve — at least temporarily. Large doses of the female sex hormones, which are produced during pregnancy, are known to help acne in any setting, but the improve-

62

ment seen in other conditions cannot be explained so easily.

A few rare skin diseases occur only during pregnancy and may represent a reaction to the developing fetus, considered an invader by the mother's immune system. A more common skin problem during pregnancy is itching. For some unfortunate women, itching begins soon after conception and remains severe until after delivery. It is harmless to both mother and child but can be a major additional stress during pregnancy. The treatments for itching discussed in Chapter 20 also apply to this situation, with the exception of antihistamine pills, since it is always unwise for a pregnant woman to use systemic drugs.

All the skin changes of pregnancy disappear within a month or two after delivery. Only an occasional stretch mark remains to remind the mother, now preoccupied with her baby, of the amazing, if temporary, transformation.

OLD AGE

Infancy begins at birth; pregnancy begins when egg meets sperm. The onset of old age has no such landmark. As discussed in the section on adulthood, it is a threshold in the gradual accumulation of damage and dysfunction — the point at which deterioration is finally all too apparent. Old age is particularly difficult to define for skin. Is skin old at age sixty-five? When the first wrinkle appears? When cuts no longer heal in a week?

From birth to death, the skin gradually changes. It   63

contains progressively less water. The cords of dermal collagen protein lose flexibility with advancing age. Elastin fibers, which give the skin its elasticity, become frayed. The epidermis thins and flattens, becomes more transparent. Melanocytes become less active and tanning ability decreases. In hair follicles, total loss of melanocyte function leads to white hair. Blood vessels in the dermis are damaged more easily — bruises appear after minor bumps and falls. The epidermal appendages — hair follicles, sweat glands, and oil glands — shrink and become less active. All over the body, hair becomes sparser and the individual hair shafts thinner. This is especially noticeable on the scalp. Oily hair becomes less oily and finally quite dry. Sweating is less profuse in hot weather or after exercise. The skin feels dry, especially in winter or in low-humidity environments. Hair and nails grow more slowly. After an injury, healing is slow and sometimes incomplete. Scars may form after injuries that formerly healed without a trace. Subcutaneous fat deposits decrease.

The combination of thinning, loss of oils and water, and altered connective tissue results in fragile, loose, wrinkled, dry skin.

In women, the hormonal changes during menopause produce additional effects in the skin. The hormone shifts cause the cutaneous blood vessels to respond erratically, and women may experience hot flashes or spontaneous sweating. The vagina becomes shorter and narrower. Its epithelial lining thins and is less resistant to injury or infection. Vaginal secretions diminish. Intercourse may become painful. Fortunately, unlike the other skin changes associated with aging, these vaginal symptoms respond to hormone therapy.

64

An estrogen cream applied directly to the vagina and surrounding skin restores the premenopausal state.

Old skin is also prone to new growths. Beginning in middle age, the skin produces a plethora of bumps and spots, most completely harmless. Each component of the skin makes its own distinctive "age spots." The epidermis makes a dime-to-quarter-sized rough raised brown or black growth called a *seborrheic keratosis*. The melanocytes generate a smooth flat brown area, usually on the face or back of the hands, called a *lentigo*. This lesion is also called a "liver spot," perhaps because of its color, since the liver plays no role in its appearance. Blood vessels contribute small bright red domes called *cherry angiomas* and slightly larger soft purple venous lakes. All these lesions are benign. A dermatologist can easily remove most of those that create a cosmetic problem, but none actually requires medical attention. Chapter 13 discusses the malignant growths that may also occur in older skin but are much less common than benign "age spots."

The changes in appearance and behavior of the skin that occur during aging are irreversible. No amount of wishing, cursing, facials, exercises, or medicated creams will restore its youthful state. The existence of a multimillion-dollar industry, built on the opposite premise, does not alter this fact. There are many excellent products that make the skin more comfortable and more attractive. Temporarily. No product slows or reverses aging.

Only one aspect of skin aging should inspire hope. It is largely preventable. Not reversible, but preventable. Chronic sun exposure is responsible for most of the wrinkling, sagging, dryness, and blotchiness of old skin. A comparison between buttock and facial skin of

65

an eighty-year-old tells the story clearly. Time itself causes some changes, but they are dwarfed by those of sun damage. No one can stop the clock, but excellent sunscreens are available to prevent sun damage. Chapter 12 discusses these products, the *only* available youth potions. In many people, skin ages faster or at least more noticeably than any other part of the body. This need not be so.

II
SKIN
PROBLEMS AND
DISEASES

9
Birthmarks, Moles, and Cysts

Developmental abnormalities are present in the skin of every person. In an organ that covers two square yards and contains millions of cells, hairs, and glands, we can expect frequent malformations. Some of these are microscopic in size and never noticed. Other malformations are large enough to be physically or emotionally incapacitating. A birthmark is a localized excess, absence, or misarrangement of the normal constituents of skin that is apparent at birth. It may form at any time during fetal development. By far the most common "birthmarks" are pigmentary alterations, such as *melanocytic nevi* — moles — and *hemangiomas* — blood vessel malformations.

There is no specific known cause for birthmarks. Intrauterine trauma seems to have no role. Certainly emotional upsets, seeing particular animals or deformed children, and other "psychic" events during the mother's pregnancy are totally without effect. Some inherited diseases are characterized by the presence of specific birthmarks, but far more often birthmarks occur in otherwise healthy children from normal families.

The skin is not the only organ with developmental abnormalities. Unimportant malformations can be found in the internal organs of most people at autopsy, but because they cannot be seen, they are rarely discovered during life.

PIGMENTED BIRTHMARKS

Moles are extremely common developmental defects that usually appear after birth, although the groundwork is laid during intrauterine life. More than 95 percent of all adults have at least one mole, and the average number is about twenty-five per person. A few are present at birth and so qualify as true birthmarks, and almost all appear before age thirty.

A mole is a clump of cells similar to melanocytes located at the base of the epidermis and/or in the dermis. Moles are usually brown or black and the same color throughout. They may be flat or raised, rough or smooth. Some have hair growing in them. Moles grow in proportion to body growth during childhood, but do not spread.

Moles themselves are harmless and require no medical attention. If it is considered unsightly, a mole may be removed surgically, although this leaves a hairline scar up to twice as long as the mole it replaces.

The concern of doctors about moles is based on the possibility of a malignant melanoma, a potentially fatal tumor, developing within them (see Chapter 13). This happens only very rarely in moles that appear after birth but is more common in congenital moles, espe-

70

cially large ones. The people at greatest risk are those with a so-called giant hairy, bathing-trunk, or *garment nevus*. As the names imply, these pigmented lesions cover large areas of the person's body and are more like clothing in texture and appearance than like skin. Melanomas arise in perhaps one in ten persons with such nevi over the course of a lifetime — bad odds indeed. Affected individuals need a complete examination, preferably by a dermatologist, at least once yearly to detect early danger signals in the skin. Fortunately, these deforming and dangerous birthmarks are quite rare. But small congenital moles are fairly common. The risk of malignancy is thousands of times less for small birthmarks, but most dermatologists still recommend surgical removal, usually a minor procedure, for moles larger than a dime. It is often easiest to do this during the first year of life, but there is no danger in waiting ten or twelve years. If trouble ever arises, it is almost always after puberty.

Mongolian spots are blue-gray, somewhat indistinct, flat areas, often on the lower back or buttocks. They are so named because they occur in virtually 100 percent of Oriental newborns. Most black babies and about 5 percent of Caucasian babies also have one or more of these spots. A Mongolian spot usually disappears slowly over several years but may never fade completely. It is made up of melanocyte-like cells in the dermis that never quite reached the epidermis during their fetal journey from the region of the brain and spinal cord (Chapter 4). Because of the skin's optical properties, the deeply buried pigment in these cells appears blue or gray rather than brown or black, as the same pigment does in the epidermal layers. The spots are completely harmless and are seldom a cosmetic concern.

HEMANGIOMAS (BLOOD VESSEL MALFORMATIONS)

Prominent hemangiomas are present in fewer than 1 percent of newborns, but minor blood vessel abnormalities of the skin can be found in most babies.

A *nevus flammeus* is a flat red or pink area present at birth. It is due to permanent dilation of otherwise normal capillaries. The most common and least noticeable type is the salmon patch or "stork bite," which is usually found at the nape of the neck or elsewhere on the head. As a rule, it fades or is covered by hair during the first year of life. More disturbing but much less frequent is the "port wine stain," a deep purple-red area that may be quite small or very large and may occur on any part of the body. It never disappears. Attempts to remove port wine stains often make their appearance worse, since a scar-producing procedure is necessary to destroy the blood vessels. Because the lesions are always completely flat, they can be masked very well by make up. Covermark® is one line of cosmetics that can be blended to match exactly the normal skin tone. Any child old enough to be embarrassed by a birthmark is old enough to use such a product.

The *strawberry hemangioma* is an initially more striking but rarely persistent blood vessel abnormality. It is sometimes present at birth but usually appears after a few weeks and then grows rapidly for several months. Parents are understandably horrified at this bright red-to-purple raised lobulated enlarging mass usually found in a conspicuous place, such as the face or neck. Virtually all parents and many physicians wish to eradicate the mark immediately by surgery, X ray, or chemical freezing. It is important to resist this tempta-

72

tion. Unlike the port wine stain, a strawberry hemangioma is composed of immature capillaries that usually involute or die out after their brief growth spurt. More than three out of four strawberry marks, no matter how large and ugly, disappear completely during childhood without any treatment, often within two to five years. Most of the rest improve considerably or heal with a small scar. Currently available treatments, on the other hand, always leave a scar and sometimes interfere with the later normal development of the treated area. In general, a strawberry hemangioma should be left alone unless it is unchanged after seven years, compromises a vital function such as eating or seeing, or causes serious bleeding problems.

CYSTS

A cyst or wen is a cavity within the skin that contains tissue fluid, cells, and cell products. Cysts may be apparent at birth but more often are first noted in adolescence or adulthood. A cyst may be quite small, detectable only as a firm bump under the skin surface, or rarely may be as large as a golf ball. Some cysts slowly enlarge over the years; most do not. Sudden enlargement usually indicates bacterial infection. Infected cysts respond rapidly to antibiotic pills but eventually return to normal even without therapy. Whatever their size, cysts are harmless and painless (except when infected).

Suspected cysts should be examined by a physician, since enlarged lymph nodes, skin cancers, and other

73

Birthmarks, Moles, and Cysts

conditions requiring medical attention are similar in appearance. Once a cyst has been diagnosed, no treatment is necessary although the lesion may be removed easily by a dermatologist or surgeon for cosmetic reasons.

Birthmarks, Moles, and Cysts

10

Chapping
and Dry Skin

Chapping is an injury to the skin produced by repeated wetting and drying. In water, skin rapidly absorbs moisture but can retain it for only a few minutes in a low-humidity environment, especially if the oil barrier on the skin surface has been removed by excessive washing (Chapter 7). The colder, drier, and windier the weather, the more rapid and extensive the water loss. The previously soft cells in the outer layers become flat and inflexible, like wood chips. Cyclic swelling and shrinking of the individual cells eventually pulls them apart. The skin becomes dry, rough, and red; if the condition is allowed to progress, painful cracks appear. Substances that normally remain on the surface can penetrate the skin and cause irritation, which magnifies the problem.

It is easier to prevent chapping than to cure it. If you are prone to chapping, wash your hands and face as infrequently as possible when the weather is cold. After washing, dry the skin surface thoroughly and immediately apply an emollient cream to the hands and lips to retard water loss. Chap Stick® or lipstick may be used on the lips. If the lips feel dry, do not lick them — apply more cream. Wear gloves when outdoors.

If your skin is already chapped, follow the same precautions even more carefully. An obviously greasy moisturizer, such as petrolatum, is more effective than a vanishing cream and may be used overnight. Thin plastic or rubber gloves or even plastic sandwich bags worn over your greased hands for several hours or overnight will speed healing. If your skin is still unimproved after a week of such care, think about consulting a dermatologist. He or she can check to be sure there is no other problem and prescribe a medicated cream or ointment to reduce inflammation.

Chapping and Dry Skin

11
Black Skin

In this chapter, we define "black skin" as skin with Negro genetic endowment, whether it is light-tan or jet-black in color. Likewise, "white skin" is skin with a Caucasian genetic background, regardless of skin tone. By these definitions, we wish to stress that many properties of skin other than its color play a role in its appearance and behavior in health and in disease.

Nearly one in eight American citizens is black, yet almost all skin care information, whether in women's magazines or doctors' offices, applies to white skin. Although white and black skin are very similar, there are enough differences to cause problems and misunderstandings in certain situations.

Black skin and white skin have the same number of pigment cells or melanocytes. As discussed in Chapter 4, the melanocytes are found in the lowest layer of the epidermis where they manufacture pigment granules and then transfer the pigment to a surrounding group of epidermal cells. Black skin is usually much darker than white skin because each pigment granule is larger, and because these pigment granules are not broken down by the body as they move upward within epidermal cells toward the skin surface. Hence, there is more melanin pigment, especially near the skin surface, in black-skinned persons.

Some of the most bothersome problems of black skin result from over- or underactivity of the pigment cells, while proportional pigment changes in white skin are usually too slight to be noticed.

Most blacks develop temporarily darkened areas when the skin is irritated in any way. Teenagers find that small pimples leave black dots that last for months, even though the pimple itself disappeared in a week. Scratches, cuts, and burns also frequently remain as dark lines or blotches long after the injury has healed. These color changes are especially distressing if they are mistaken for permanent scars. The best treatment for this *postinflammatory hyperpigmentation*, as it is called by dermatologists, is prevention. Acne, for example, may be treated vigorously with antibiotics to prevent the lesions from appearing (see Chapter 23). Nervous habits of rubbing or picking at skin must be controlled. Antihistamine medication may be prescribed to minimize itchy sensations in conditions such as eczema, so that scratching can be avoided (see Chapter 20). Once a dark spot is present, it should be left alone! Touching and rubbing will just encourage the melanocytes to make more pigment. Bleach creams that contain hydroquinone such as Artra®, Eldoquin®, and Esoterica® will help lighten the area, but this bleaching can take several weeks or even months to make a difference.

After a mild injury, the pigment cells in black skin may temporarily become less active than their normal, undisturbed neighbors so that light spots appear which may last for months. Often the "injury" is so mild that

78

it goes unnoticed, and the change in color is the only evidence. Dermatologists call this condition *pityriasis alba*, meaning white flaky area, although the flakiness or scaling is sometimes unapparent. These pale areas are seen most often in children and usually affect the cheeks or upper arms. They are harmless and temporary. Most children seem to outgrow the condition by adolescence. If the color difference embarrasses the child, a dermatologist can prescribe a steroid cream to hasten recovery.

Vitiligo, a fairly common skin disease in both blacks and whites, is fully discussed in Chapter 14. It is mentioned here not only to point out that loss of pigment is more disfiguring in blacks than in whites, but also to stress the fact that it is completely different from pityriasis alba. When pigment is suppressed by injury or inflammation, the skin appears lighter than normal, but never absolutely white, as in vitiligo, and the change is always reversible, while in vitiligo the normal color returns only in some patients and only after prolonged treatment. A condition with permanent loss of pigmentation, nearly identical to vitiligo, can be produced by applying certain chemicals such as monobenzylether of hydroquinone (not to be confused with hydroquinone) to the skin in order to lighten its color. Such products may be advertised as producing partial, uniform loss of pigment desired by some dark-skinned persons. Unfortunately, as many black people, especially in Africa, have learned from personal experience, they can also cause permanent total pigment loss in confettilike spots on large areas. In America today all "bleaching creams" are tested before appearing on the market. Products containing hydroquinone, for example, are safe and effective when used as directed to lighten skin color and are sometimes prescribed by dermatologists to reverse hyperpigmentation, as discussed above.

A reaction characteristic primarily of black skin is seen in many patients with eczema. In areas that are frequently itchy and hence scratched or rubbed, the skin not only may darken but may also develop innumerable small bumps resembling insect bites. This is called *papular lichenification*. Both black and white patients with eczema frequently develop "standard" lichenification, which is a thickening of the skin with prominent skin markings. The papular or bumpy type occurs almost exclusively in blacks. The bumps are a direct result of rubbing or scratching; they always go away after several weeks when the rubbing stops. A doctor may prescribe a topical steroid cream to sooth the skin and antihistamine pills to reduce the tendency to scratch or rub unconsciously.

Another rather common problem in black skin is abnormal scarring. *Keloids* are firm, raised, rubbery masses of scar tissue that continue to grow after the original wound is repaired. Keloids may occur after very minor skin injuries but are more common in surgical scars or major wounds. No one knows why they occur. There is no way to predict whether the skin of a certain individual will form keloids, but black skin is, in general, quite susceptible, and if a keloid scar has already occurred, the risk of further keloid formation is probably increased. People are most likely to develop keloids in late childhood and early adulthood. Small children and elderly people rarely do. This means that elective surgery, such as removing a birthmark, might, for example, be done earlier rather than later in childhood or a hernia repair operation might be postponed from age thirty to age forty if there are no symptoms.

As with hyperpigmentation, prevention is the best treatment. It is wise to avoid such unnecessary skin injuries as ear piercing. If an injury does occur or an operation must be done, the physician should be alerted about any predisposition to form keloid scars. In people at high risk, the injured area of skin may be injected with steroids and even treated with X rays at intervals until healing is complete. Such procedures usually (but not always) prevent keloid formation. They are not appropriate for every patient but may be helpful, especially when a keloid scar is being removed surgically for cosmetic reasons.

More common, but less bothersome and easier to treat, is a condition called *dermatosis papulosa nigra*, a Latin locution meaning bumpy black rash. Beginning in adolescence or early adulthood, many blacks develop numerous dark brown or black raised pinpoint spots on the face. They are neither itchy nor painful but if numerous can be cosmetically annoying. These harmless lesions also occur commonly in whites but less often on the face and rarely before the sixth decade. They can be easily removed by a dermatologist, usually without leaving any visible scar.

Some problems of black skin are related to tightly curly or kinky hair. Black men are sometimes plagued by an itchy, bumpy rash in the beard area where they shave. Dermatologists call this *sycosis barbae*. When the beard is shaved, the tips of hair remaining at the skin surface are sharp. As the hairs grow out, the tips curl back toward the skin surface and actually puncture it. The skin responds to this injury just as it would to a splinter: the area becomes red, slightly swollen, and tender or itchy. The area may also darken in color. As more hairs are involved, the skin surface becomes very irregular and more difficult to shave, compounding the problem. There is a simple cure—stop shaving. Once the hairs are long, it is easy for them to curl back away from the skin surface; no new lesions will appear. For men who don't want a beard, the solution is somewhat more complicated. An electric shaver is helpful because it makes a blunter tip on the beard hairs than a razor blade. A men's depilatory such as Magic Shave®, which dissolves the hairs chemically, when used according to directions, is even better. Finally, a mild steroid cream may be prescribed by your doctor to relieve the existing lesions. It must be remembered, however, that prolonged use of a steroid cream on the face is never advisable.

The styling and grooming of black hair may create insidious problems. Hair damage or loss may be so gradual or delayed in onset that the person cannot believe there is a simple cause and effect relationship. In the past, hot combing and hair straightening with harsh chemicals caused temporary or permanent hair loss in many men and women. More recently, the practice of braiding hair very tightly in cornrows has produced loss of hair due to a constant pull on the root. Such hair loss is usually most prominent along the parts, which seem to widen. At first, the hair is still able to regrow, but eventually the root is destroyed and the hair loss is permanent. Some people are able to braid their hair for many years before such damage is seen. Probably there is no harm in putting such stress on hair as long as it continues to grow normally. But once areas of baldness appear, another hair style should be chosen. A true Afro is a very healthy style for black hair, but vigorous back combing will break the hair shafts.

A final, positive note: black skin is virtually immune to sun damage. Aging black skin remains smooth, firm, and youthful-looking. The aging changes of wrinkling, dryness, and blotchy pigmentation that appear in many whites by the fourth decade are rarely seen before the seventh decade in blacks. Skin cancer, which accounts for more than half of the cancers in white patients, is almost nonexistent in blacks.

12
Fair Skin

A fair complexion has long been valued in Western society and like most prized possessions, it requires careful maintenance. The blond or redheaded beauty of eighteen too often develops dry, coarsened skin before the age of forty and skin cancers before the age of fifty.

What is fair skin? Natural blonds and redheads, especially those with blue eyes, are usually considered to have a fair complexion. Some classify complexion according to the pallor of untanned skin, regardless of hair and eye color. The best standard for judging fair skin, however, at least in terms of its *vulnerability*, is its reaction to the sun. A person with platinum hair, blue eyes, and pale skin who tans evenly is less fair-skinned than a brunette who freckles and burns. People with similar "coloring" may have very different risks of developing long-term permanent sun damage. Whether a person sunburns or suntans after a single sun exposure seems to be a reliable indicator of this risk. Whites may be classified into four "Skin Types," ranging from very susceptible (Type I) to very resistant (Type IV) with respect to skin cancer and premature aging

TABLE OF SKIN TYPES

Skin Type	Response to sun (first 30-minute exposure of the summer)	Protection recommended	Preparation recommended Clear lotion	Milky lotion	Cream
I	Always burns; never tans	Daily sunscreen	Pabanol®	Piz Buin (protective tanning lotion) Number 6®	Piz Buin Exclusiv Extrem Number 6®
II	Usually burns; sometimes tans faintly	Sunscreens for all intentional sun exposures	PreSun® Paba-Gel®	Eclipse®	
III	Sometimes burns; usually tans	Sunscreen for protracted sun exposure	Block-Out® Pabafilm®		
IV	Never burns; always tans well	None necessary			

changes, based on the expected reaction to a first hypothetical thirty-minute summer sun exposure (see the table).

The curse of fair skin is sun exposure. The first problem encountered by a fair-skinned person is repeated, sometimes severe, sunburns. Each burn is painful, and ease of sunburning may limit outdoor activities in sunny climates.

The second problem is freckling. Freckles are a desperate attempt by the skin to form a protective pigment layer when it is being damaged by sun. In people with fair skin, especially those with Celtic ancestry, small groups of heroic pigment cells become permanently overactive, forming freckles, while the areas between freckles remain unprotected. Freckles are considered cute in children, but many teenagers and adults find them a cosmetic liability. More important, freckles are a warning.

Other problems may not appear for many years, but often surface in early middle age. Chronically sun-exposed skin in areas such as the face and back of the hands becomes dry, loose, and wrinkled. Small red lines — dilated blood vessels — appear on the face and neck, then on other areas as well (see Chapter 19). The neck and chest develop a pebbly texture. Pigmentation becomes more irregular and "age spots" appear. The skin looks old. After another decade or so, skin tumors may begin to appear (see Chapter 13) and gradually enlarge unless treatment is provided. These changes inexorably progress despite the use of moisturizers, skin toners, facials, and hormone creams.

What can be done? Sun damage begins in infancy, the first time you go outdoors. It is cumulative and irreversible. Changes produced by a sunburn do not disappear when the peeling stops. Sun exposures too brief to result in sunburn also cause some damage. Even if the skin still looks unchanged after ten or twenty years of sunbathing, much damage has occurred. Under the microscope, collagen proteins in the dermis appear fragmented. If sun exposure continues, these microscopic protein alterations eventually cause sagging and wrinkling of the skin surface. While sunlight slowly destroys the skin's supporting fibers, it also damages living cells in the epidermis above. For many years the body is able to repair these injuries, but eventually the repair process is overwhelmed and abnormal cells persist. These cells form cancers.

Protection from the sun ideally should begin at birth. Practically speaking, it should begin *now*.

It is not necessary to forfeit outdoor activities. The most damaging wavelengths of sunlight penetrate the atmosphere to a limited extent. They reach the earth's surface in significant amounts only at midday (10 A.M. to 2 P.M.) and in temperate climates only during spring and summer. Avoiding midday sun reduces solar damage considerably.

The best protection from unwanted sun exposure is regular use of effective sunscreens. Several excellent products are available in most drugstores, but the most popular and widely advertised sunscreens are not sufficient for people with Skin Types I and II. Lotions and creams that contain para-aminobenzoic acid (PABA) are often reliable protectors, but some new formulations are far superior to others. Only recently have a few companies begun to determine the precise degree of protection afforded by their sunscreen products (see table). Federal regulatory agencies are concerned that sunscreen users at present cannot learn from the label whether the product is minimally or maximally effective, or indeed totally misrepresented. For example, so-called tanning lotions are purchased and used by thousands of people in the belief they aid the tanning process, whereas in fact only ultraviolet light can cause tanning and no product can hasten tanning while avoiding sunburn. The table suggests several sunscreen brands for Skin Types I and II that have been proved capable of blocking at least ten sunburn doses of sunlight in fair-skinned people. That is, if a burn normally occurs after a thirty-minute exposure, more than five hours are necessary for the same reaction when the sunscreen is used. Additional precautions are needed for highly sensitive areas such as the nose and lips during protracted exposures. A plastic nose guard attached to sunglasses affords excellent protection, but if this is too cumbersome, an opaque sunscreen containing zinc oxide or titanium oxide provides virtually complete protection for the nose. Zinc oxide ointment, U.S.P., is the best, but needs to be applied so thickly that the nose looks white. For the lips, zinc oxide ointment again is the best, but good protection can be obtained with RVPABA® lipstick or Uval® sunstick.

Sunscreens should be applied to all exposed areas at least twenty minutes before going into the sunlight. Very fair-skinned people (Types I and II), especially those in tropical or subtropical climates, should apply a sunscreen lotion (see table) every day as part of their morning routine, since repeated brief, unplanned sun exposures occur all day. Making six trips to the car, taking in the wash, and briefly weeding the garden can lead to a sunburn as severe as that following two hours of deliberate sunbathing. Sunscreens must be reapplied after washing, swimming, or heavy sweating.

Wearing wide-brimmed hats or sitting under a beach umbrella is a poor substitute for using a sunscreen. Skin protected in such ways receives at least half the amount of sun damage that totally unprotected skin does, since much sunlight is reflected onto the face and body from the ground and other surfaces around us. Hazy or cloudy days also fail to prevent sunburn. Up to 80 percent of the ultraviolet (sunburn) rays may reach the earth's surface on such days. The risk of accidental overexposure is probably increased compared with that on sunny days, because clouds and haze do absorb the infrared (heat) rays that usually cause people to curtail their sunbathing. Severe sunburns can also occur in midwinter, despite the greatly reduced ultraviolet intensity of sunlight in that season. Skiers and other snow-sport enthusiasts are the usual victims, since fresh snow is an excellent reflector and nearly doubles one's sun exposure.

Many people view sunscreens as an unwelcome interloper in their communion with nature. Sunscreens evoke the same reactions among sun worshipers as condoms do among young lovers. Unfortunately, at this time there is no pill that prevents sun damage. People who find a mechanical barrier too oppressive must accept the consequences. They take longer than nine months, but premature aging changes do eventually appear in chronically sun-exposed fair skin.

For many years, dark tans have been in vogue. This was not always the case, however. From ancient times through the aristocracies of nineteenth-century Europe, men and women of fashion carefully protected themselves from the sun. White skin was the ideal. This standard probably reflected the fact that tanning was associated with the rural working classes who were forced to be outdoors much of the time. Perhaps the lords and ladies were also astute enough to notice that the sun-exposed skin of their peasants aged much more rapidly than their own. In any case, fashion has reversed itself. A year-round tan now connotes wealth and leisure time, the beautiful people. For those with a dark complexion (Types III and IV), pursuit of a tan is a relatively harmless pastime. For fair-skinned people (Types I and II), repeated efforts to coax a tan from their ill-equipped pigment cells are nothing short of self-destruction.

Fair Skin

13
Skin Cancer

Cancer is a bad word. Virtually everyone is afraid of it, and for most people it is the worst imaginable illness. Yet, like almost all biologic processes, cancer is a spectrum. At one end of the spectrum, it is a killer, but at the other pole it is sometimes little more than an annoyance and a cosmetic problem.

Cancer implies a disorderly proliferation of cells that no longer respond to the normal controls of the body — cells that have lost the concept of "enough." Cancerous cells rarely divide faster than their normal counterparts, but divide endlessly and hence eventually require more than their share of space in the body. When cancer cells leave their original site and usurp space in the lungs, brain, liver, or other vital organs, they may impair normal functions and cause death. Some cancers spread when they are still microscopic in size; others never do.

Individual cells in a cancer are usually quite abnormal in appearance as well as in behavior. This feature allows a doctor to recognize a cancer under the microscope at any time, even before it has spread to other parts of the body or has invaded the surrounding normal tissues. Unfortunately, it is impossible to obtain tissue of an entire person for microscopic examination at judicious time intervals, in order to detect cancers before they grow and spread. For most organs of the body, early detection of cancer remains an elusive goal.

A skin cancer differs from other cancers in the same way that the skin differs from other organs: you can see it. Most internal cancers go undiscovered for years, until they become large enough to be felt through many layers of fat and muscle or until they interfere with normal functioning of other body parts. Conversely, a trained physician can find and diagnose most skin cancers when they are less than ⅛ inch in diameter. Indeed, most people first become aware of new skin growths on their own body surface at about this size, although they may not be concerned enough to seek a medical opinion. Once suspected, a skin cancer can easily be biopsied for microscopic confirmation and then be treated. The visibility of these tumors is a major factor in the highly favorable outlook for people with skin cancer.

Until the late 1940s, it was believed that exposure to the sun promoted health. The more sun exposure, the better. In recent years, as sun worshiping became a national pastime, its dangers came more clearly into focus. A single fifteen-minute exposure to the summer sun can produce sunburn. For approximately two-thirds of the white population, those with Skin Types III and IV (see Chapter 12), repeated sun exposures result in a protective tan. But in fair-skinned people, those with Skin Types I and II, little or no protective tanning occurs. Repeated exposures lead to repeated sunburns and progressive damage.

92　　　　The most serious effect of overexposure to the sun is

the development of skin cancer. There are three major types: *basal cell carcinoma, squamous cell carcinoma,* and *malignant melanoma.*

BASAL AND SQUAMOUS CELL CARCINOMAS

These two types of skin cancer considered together are the most frequently detected of all cancers in man. Fortunately, they are also the most easily and most successfully treated and account for less than 0.1 percent of cancer deaths.

The evidence implicating chronic sun exposure in the development of basal and squamous cell cancers is irrefutable. The great majority occur on the parts of the body most exposed to sun: the face, tips of the ears (in men), and backs of the hands. They are most frequently seen in farmers, ranchers, sailors, construction men and other outdoor workers, in sports enthusiasts and others who pursue year-round outdoor recreation. These cancers are also more common in sunny climates. In the United States, the South and Southwest report many more cases than do the northern states. Finally, fair-skinned people are much more likely to be affected than their darker-skinned neighbors and co-workers.

Basal and squamous cell carcinomas usually appear as tiny ulcers that do not heal or as small firm, flesh-colored bumps with fine blood vessels laced over their surfaces. They grow very slowly and often appear unchanged for months or even years. Lesions first noticed after age forty or fifty are most suspicious.

If you are fair-complexioned (Skin Type I or II),

93

spend many hours outdoors, and especially if you live in a sunny climate, it is very likely that you already have or will eventually develop a basal or squamous cell carcinoma.

What can you do to prevent skin cancer and what should you do if you are already affected?

Daily use of an effective sunscreen (Chapter 12) is the most important preventive measure. Annual examinations of the skin surface for early cancers or precancerous lesions are very helpful for high-risk individuals after age forty. These measures are especially important for people who have already had a basal cell or squamous cell carcinoma, since they have a one in three chance every year of developing a new skin cancer.

A relatively small number of basal and squamous cell carcinomas are not related to past sun exposure. Rarely, they can be attributed to one of several inherited conditions. Many have occurred and continue to occur as the result of two practices that were common in the first half of this century: ingestion of arsenic, which was found in "spring tonics" and various medications such as Fowler's solution and on unwashed farm produce as an insecticide; and exposure to X rays either inadvertently, at work, or through treatment for skin diseases such as acne or ringworm infection of the scalp. We now know that even short courses of X ray, once used to treat thousands of patients and believed safe at the time, produce permanent skin changes and sometimes even skin cancers many years later. If you were ever exposed to arsenic or X rays, you should have a yearly examination to detect developing skin cancers. People with prior X-ray therapy for acne or scalp ringworm can also be checked at this time for evidence of thyroid cancer, a

much less common but more serious aftereffect of ir-
radiation to the head and neck.

If you think you may have a skin cancer, see your
general physician or dermatologist promptly. Overall,
95 percent of these tumors are cured by a single treatment such as surgical excision, X ray, or freezing with
liquid nitrogen. However, the larger the lesion, the
larger the scar after treatment and the greater the risk
of recurrence.

MALIGNANT MELANOMA

Malignant melanomas, also called melanomas, are
life-threatening hazards of sun exposure. They are as
common among whites as Hodgkin's disease or primary malignant brain tumors. Only two-thirds of melanoma patients survive for five years, about the same
survival rate as for breast cancer patients. Melanomas
are the leading cause of death of all diseases arising in
the skin. Each year there are 8,000 new cases in the
United States and 2,800 of these new patients die
within five years.

The cause of most melanomas is unknown, just as it
is for most malignancies of any kind. However, sun
exposure, which normally incites melanocytes to divide during the tanning process, is at least partially responsible for their malignant conversion in certain
cases. Like basal and squamous cell carcinomas, melanomas are more common in people living in the lower
latitudes. They occur more frequently in fair-skinned
people than in those who tan well and are rare in
blacks — although not as rare, relatively, as basal and

95

squamous cell carcinomas. Similarly, while melanoma does not occur most frequently on the most exposed areas of the body, neither does it occur frequently on the least exposed areas (such as those covered by a bathing suit or by long pants in men). Unlike the other skin cancers, which occur in people with outdoor occupations and regular sun exposure, melanoma tends to strike professional and managerial workers who have intermittent sun exposure during weekends and vacations. And it occurs in body sites that traditionally have been concealed but are increasingly being exposed because of altered modes of dress. Very recent analyses of melanoma in Norway show that the rate of increase for melanoma of the skin between 1955 and 1975 was even larger than that for lung cancer. This striking increase is attributed to longer vacations with easy transportation to sunny areas. The increased incidence of melanoma in the United States also is believed to be related to changes in life-styles that have occurred since World War II: more leisure time, more money for travel to Florida or to the Caribbean during winter months, and to a great extent the new mystique that has developed about tanned skin. In the nineteenth century, the aristocracy sought cameo-white complexions. Ladies wore long skirts and wide-brimmed hats and used parasols (literally, "for the sun"). But changing styles have dictated less and less clothing for sports and recreation: rising hemlines, bikinis, shorts. Melanomas are now appearing in just these newly exposed areas: the upper backs of both sexes and the lower legs of women. And melanomas are occurring in younger and younger people, most commonly those between twenty-five and fifty years old.

96   What can be done to prevent melanoma?

Because sun damage may contribute to the development of melanoma, sunscreens are theoretically helpful but would not be expected to offer dramatic protection as in the case of basal cell and squamous cell carcinoma. Some physicians recommend surgical removal of pigmented birthmarks, since approximately one melanoma in four arises in such a lesion. Unfortunately, the highest risk is for people with very large birthmarks (see Chapter 9) that are usually impossible to remove completely. People with very large pigmented birthmarks should be examined annually for evidence of early malignant change. There is little justification for removing moles that first appear during childhood or early adulthood, since the average person has about twenty-five (some have hundreds), and the risk of malignant change for any one mole is exceedingly small.

Early detection is the key to successful treatment of melanoma. Thousands of lives could be saved each year if these malignancies were recognized and removed before they had time to spread. There are five danger signals for a mole or other pigmented skin lesion. First, melanomas are multicolored. Melanomas often contain areas of red, white, and blue or at least several shades of brown to jet-black. Benign lesions may be any of these colors but rarely have a mixture of different colors. Second, melanomas have irregular borders, often with a notch. Benign lesions usually have a smooth, regular border. Third, there are raised areas within a generally flat pigmented spot. Melanomas often have an irregular surface resembling a topographic map, rather than a uniformly raised or uniformly flat surface. A fourth sign is rapid growth, and the fifth, easy bleeding. Any of these five signs is a good reason to have the suspicious area examined by an experienced physician. If the doctor is not completely sure the lesion is harmless, a small biopsy always reveals the correct diagnosis.

Once a melanoma is diagnosed, it should be treated promptly at an appropriate facility. Such referrals need never take more than a week. Major centers offer the best hope of cure. After the melanoma has been removed, such centers also assure appropriate checkups and can provide further treatment if necessary.

The treatment of early melanoma consists of excising the lesion plus a border of normal tissue and sometimes the adjacent lymph nodes. In more advanced cases, use of cancer chemotherapy or special vaccinations to increase the body's immune defenses are also recommended. Mutilating operations, such as amputation of a limb, are virtually never necessary.

Skin cancer does not deserve the same reputation as other cancers. The most common types can be prevented and, failing that, are almost always curable. All skin cancers are best managed by prompt diagnosis and treatment. But you must take the initiative. It is your skin. No one is closer to it than you yourself.

14

Pigment Loss (Vitiligo)

Approximately 1 percent of the world's population — more than 30 million people — has *vitiligo*. The name vitiligo comes from the Latin word for defect or blemish. Medically, vitiligo means that certain areas of skin and sometimes hair lose all their pigmentation and appear white. The melanocytes or pigment-producing cells seem to vanish from affected areas. The skin is otherwise normal and no other part of the body is affected. Without treatment, the pigment loss is almost always permanent. The process can begin at any age and in most cases gradually involves more and more of the skin surface. Men and women are equally affected. Certain patterns of involvement are more common, but any part of the body may become white and some people ultimately lose all their pigmentation. The most common pattern is symmetrical — for each white spot on the left side of the body, there is a mirror-image spot on the right side. Bony areas, such as the knees, ankles, and knuckles, are favored. White rings around the mouth and eyes and genitals also occur frequently. Rarely, the hair may lose its pigmentation; only the iris of the eye is never affected.

If a person with vitiligo injures normally pigmented skin, that area may lose its pigment as it heals. For example, a modest cut may be replaced by a permanent white line.

The cause of vitiligo is unknown, but some evidence suggests an "autoimmune" etiology. Body defense mechanisms that usually attack germs and other alien substances begin to attack normal body cells — the melanocytes. People with vitiligo and their relatives seem to have some propensity to other autoimmune diseases as well, especially those that affect the thyroid gland. Only a few people with vitiligo have other medical problems, however, and these can be detected by a medical examination.

A relatively minor problem for vitiligo skin is easy sunburn. The white areas have no natural protection from the sun and may repeatedly burn, blister, and peel, while the normal skin tans. Regular use of an effective sunscreen (see Chapter 12) is the answer.

Although vitiligo does not impair health in any way, it can be a crippling cosmetic problem. This is especially true for dark-skinned people in whom the white spots are most obvious. Vitiligo can be a personal tragedy. Some of the "lepers" mentioned in the Bible had vitiligo, and even today in some societies people with vitiligo are outcasts.

A person with vitiligo has several options. First, he or she can do nothing. The condition is harmless and cannot be transmitted to others. In fair-skinned people, the white spots may be virtually impossible to distinguish from the normal skin color except with a special examining light. If spots become noticeable in the summer because of tanning in pigmented areas, a sunscreen can be used to block the tanning.

100   A second option is to use either a makeup or dye on

the white spots. This may be preferable for a person with a small area of involvement or one who is bothered by the spots only on "special" occasions. Several cosmetic manufacturers, such as Lydia O'Leary who makes Covermark®, will exactly match a liquid makeup to the normal skin color. A single daily application can make the vitiligo invisible. The disadvantages are clear: makeup washes off with swimming or sweating; it must be fastidiously applied; and if the normal skin is allowed to tan, at least one additional makeup shade is needed. Skin dyes (chemicals that stain the top layer of the skin or stratum corneum) are effective until this skin layer is shed, usually in three to five days. To be sure, this eliminates the problem of the dye's washing off, but unfortunately, only a few shades are available, and often the dyed areas differ slightly from the normal skin color. Dyes are even more difficult to apply than makeup, because if the normally pigmented skin at the edge of a spot is not completely shielded, it also will stain and form a dark halo.

A third option is to attempt actual repigmentation of the white areas. This treatment requires detailed instruction and supervision by an experienced physician. Many doctors are unfamiliar with vitiligo and may not even know that a treatment is available. An expert should always be consulted initially, if possible. In this process, a medication called *psoralen* (pronounced sōr-a-len) is taken by mouth, or in special cases applied to the involved skin surface, and the patient is then exposed either to sunlight or to a special type of artificial ultraviolet light. Each treatment takes a few minutes to several hours, depending on many factors, and is repeated two or three times weekly for many months for well over one hundred treatments. The treatment is

101

safe when done correctly, but cure is by no means guaranteed. It is obvious that a person must be highly motivated to undergo this therapy. When vitiligo begins early in life, it is usually wise to defer treatment until the child is old enough to be bothered by his appearance and so wish to cooperate with the regimen. There is no harm in waiting. Vitiligo responds equally well to treatment whether it has been present for months or for many years, and treating existing spots will not prevent new spots from appearing in the future. Despite the drawbacks, many people have dramatic, often permanent return of normal pigmentation after sufficient treatment. It is always worthwhile at least to discuss the possibility of treatment with a doctor who can estimate your chances of benefiting from this kind of program and answer your specific questions.

The fourth option is for patients with very extensive vitiligo. Depigmenting the remaining normal skin can be a relatively simple solution to a difficult problem. When the entire skin surface is white, the appearance is quite satisfactory. Many patients receive compliments on their alabaster skin from unsuspecting friends. Depigmentation also requires prescription medication, a cream that destroys pigment cells, and careful supervision by an experienced physician. The process usually requires nine to twelve months. It is irreversible. If a cure for vitiligo is discovered tomorrow, it will not help patients who have undergone chemical depigmentation.

Vitiligo is a complicated and discouraging condition, but by no means hopeless. Effective treatment is already available, and the future is promising.

Pigment Loss (Vitiligo)

15
Dandruff

The skin of the scalp is constantly replacing itself, creating new cells at the bottom and shedding dead cells at the surface. In this way, it is like skin all over the body. If large numbers of cells in the dead upper layer are shed together as white "flakes" rather than as inconspicuous single cells, you have dandruff. Oils are produced by glands associated with hair follicles and undoubtedly trap some shedding cells in dandruff scales, but the exact cause of this common problem is unknown.

There is no cure for dandruff. It is as easy to change the color of your eyes as to change the behavior of your scalp. However, in virtually all cases, dandruff can be controlled; the scalp will appear normal as long as treatment is continued.

The first step toward control of dandruff is frequent shampooing. There is no danger in washing the hair and scalp even every day, as long as the soap is thoroughly rinsed out. On the other hand, there is no benefit in washing more often than necessary to eradicate scales. It is helpful to use a shampoo specially formulated for dandruff control. Such shampoos contain zirconium, salicylic acid, sulfur, or other substances that lessen the formation of new scales and allow existing scales to be rinsed off the scalp surface during the shampoo. Tar shampoos for dandruff control are also available without prescription. They are more effective than the first group, but, as you might imagine, are messy to use. They look, feel, and smell like tar, and may stain blond or gray hair.

If dandruff persists despite frequent use of a medicated shampoo, consider visiting a dermatologist or other doctor interested in skin disorders. In many cases, your doctor can suggest specific shampoos or prescribe a steroid-containing lotion to use once or twice daily on your scalp to stop the scaling. People with severe dandruff often have an underlying skin problem, such as seborrheic dermatitis (Chapter 29) or psoriasis (Chapter 24) and have much to gain from a dermatologic consultation.

The special case of severe dandruff in infants is called "cradle cap." Scales build up on the scalp, and may temporarily interfere with hair growth. This condition causes no permanent damage. Cradle cap always disappears and rarely lasts more than a few months, but it is sometimes a sign that the child will have seborrheic dermatitis or psoriasis later in life. Babies are more attractive and probably more comfortable if the scales are removed as thoroughly as possible. Rub mineral oil into the baby's scalp, wait a few hours, then gently comb or pick out the scales, and shampoo thoroughly. If this regimen is unsuccessful, your pediatrician or dermatologist can prescribe medications to remove the scales.

Dandruff can affect the eyebrows, eyelashes, and chest hair as well as the scalp. Steroid-containing creams or lotions, prescribed by your doctor, can control it.

104

16
Hair Loss

Loss of hair can be psychologically devastating. The mere possibility of hair loss is a significant concern for some people. Once in a great while, hair loss is an indication of physical illness, as well as a social and cosmetic problem, and hence doubly worrisome.

Each of us loses approximately one hundred scalp hairs daily in the normal process of hair growth cycles (see Chapter 5). These hairs are quickly replaced by new ones. True hair loss is also part of normal aging. In many men and most women, the process is subtle and has no cosmetic or medical significance. This chapter deals with hair loss that is disturbing to the affected person either in extent or location. Baldness is the best-known example, but many other conditions can produce temporary or permanent hair loss.

BALDNESS (NORMAL HAIR LOSS)

Baldness is difficult to define. To one person it means total absence of scalp hair; to another it means a hairline receding at the temples. There is no precise medical definition. For our purposes, baldness is an exaggeration of the normal process of hair loss (see Chapter 5) that is sufficient to cause a person embarrassment or to alter his self-image.

Baldness is not really hair loss, in fact, but a change in the type of hair present on the scalp: previously long, thick hairs are replaced by extremely thin short ones that are barely visible without a magnifying glass. This change in hair type occurs gradually and in a predictable pattern on the scalp. The exact reasons why people become bald are not known, but hereditary and hormonal factors are certainly involved.

There are two problems associated with baldness: worrying about whether you will go bald and wondering what to do about it if you are bald.

First, only men go bald. Women never lose so much hair in the process of balding that they appear hairless. In the most extreme case, a woman may experience marked thinning of the scalp hair, to the extent that she has difficulty concealing her scalp with certain hair styles. This degree of hair loss is understandably upsetting, and hence fits our original definition of baldness, but in women the process is never complete. In addition, balding is slower in women than in men and is rarely noticeable before the seventh decade even in severe cases. Significant hair loss in younger women is almost always due to something other than routine baldness and should be evaluated by an experienced physician, preferably a dermatologist.

About 10 percent of men develop baldness in a way that women do not. This difference is due primarily to high levels of the male sex hormone testosterone (androgen). It must be stressed, however, that neither men nor women go bald because of hormone imbalance. The normal presence of testosterone in men simply encourages a genetically determined process to occur. Which men will go bald? Often, baldness runs in families. If your father or other male relatives are bald, your chance of extensive, early hair loss is high. However, it is possible for only one male in a family to inherit all the genes necessary for baldness, or for some males to avoid this inheritance. A bald father may have sons whose hair is still thick at age sixty; a young man rapidly losing his hair may complain that his father, brothers, uncles, and grandfathers all have full heads of hair. Once hair loss has begun, a prediction about eventual baldness can be made with more confidence, however. Men who are destined to have extensive hair loss usually notice a receding hairline and thinning of hair on the top of the head during their twenties or occasionally earlier. In general, the earlier hair loss appears and the faster it progresses, the worse the outlook. A forty-year-old man who detects some thinning while washing his hair should not worry about impending baldness!

What can be done for baldness?

Magazine advertisements and drugstores offer a plethora of miracle creams and pills, but these treatments do not alter the fact of baldness. Hair loss is permanent. There is no way to restore the tiny residual hairs to their former thickness and length. At the present time, there is no cure and no prevention for baldness — it is best to accept that fact. Toupees and wigs have been used throughout history and for some people are well worth the inconvenience and potential embarrassment. Such hair pieces are available in all styles and all price ranges; many are impossible to detect on casual inspection.

In recent years, hair transplantation has been publicized as a "breakthrough." It is a long-term and

107

expensive proposition. During each visit, the dermatologist or surgeon numbs an area of the scalp with injections of a local anesthetic. Using a circular blade that resembles a small cookie cutter, the doctor then removes ten to one hundred skin plugs from that part of the scalp with the most dense hair growth. Each plug of skin is about 1/6 inch in diameter and contains three or four hairs. An equal number of plugs are removed from the bald scalp and hair-bearing plugs are fitted into the holes. The hairless plugs are discarded, and the holes in the donor area of the scalp gradually shrink down and form inconspicuous scars. Usually several hundred plugs must be transplanted over a period of time to correct moderately advanced baldness. If the operation is done properly (and often it is not), the transplanted hairs live and resume normal growth. When the hair is properly groomed, the appearance is quite natural. Hair transplantation has many advocates among patients and doctors, but, at a cost of several months' time and several thousand dollars, it should not be undertaken lightly. Moreover, not everyone is a candidate, even if he can afford the time and money. If baldness is very extensive, there is no donor area from which to obtain hair-bearing plugs. This problem cannot be avoided by transplantation early in life — if hairs are transplanted from an area destined to become bald later in life, the hairs disappear at the fated time, no matter where they are grafted.

There is no truly satisfactory solution to the problem of baldness. Still, a person distraught by baldness or its specter should not hesitate to seek medical help. Often a person's fear of future baldness is unfounded; occasionally the hair loss is not due to baldness but to another, perhaps treatable, condition. In many cases,

108

simply discussing the facts with a knowledgeable person is beneficial.

ALOPECIA AREATA

In *alopecia areata*, certain areas of the body, usually on the scalp, suddenly lose all their hair. This condition differs from baldness in that the hair loss is sudden, patchy but complete within the involved areas, and reversible; it affects men and women equally and is more common in children than in adults.

Often overnight, and without warning, a dime- or quarter-sized bald spot appears. The spot is totally hairless but otherwise normal. There is no pain, itching, or rash. The affected person feels well; only the hair is involved. Once a spot appears it usually remains unchanged for several months and then, again for no apparent reason, the hair regrows. Often several spots appear over a period of weeks to months. Individual spots may enlarge before hair regrowth begins and hairs at the edge of a spot may fall out easily when brushed or pulled.

There may be only one episode in a lifetime, or spots may come and go for years. An episode may consist of a single small bald spot, easily covered by the adjacent normal hair, or may involve extensive hair loss. Rarely, all the hair is lost.

Regardless of the amount or duration of hair loss, alopecia areata is always reversible. All the empty hair follicles are capable of again producing normal hair, and almost all eventually do even without treatment.

109

Hair Loss

As with many disorders, it is easier to state what does *not* cause alopecia areata than what does. It is not an infection or allergy; it is not hereditary or contagious. In some cases alopecia areata is a response to severe emotional upset or stress. Such stresses may be difficult for the person involved to recognize or admit and may not be obvious even to family members or close friends. At times, however, no cause can be found for this mysterious disorder.

A dermatologist or other physician familiar with hair disorders can usually diagnose alopecia areata immediately. Often the doctor can make a rough prediction of the future course, based on the amount and pattern of hair loss and age at which the problem began. Treatment is rarely indicated, but in extensive or persistent cases, a dermatologist may recommend steroid medication in the form of creams or injections for the hairless areas. Steroid pills should not be used, however, since the risks are unjustified and the results of such therapy too often disappointing. If emotional factors appear to play a role, psychiatric consultation may be requested. If hair cannot be made to regrow, a wig or other form of hair substitute should be considered. Unfortunately, hair transplantation is not an option, since the transplanted area usually also develops alopecia areata.

The family and friends of a person with alopecia areata often exert a strong influence on the course of the disorder. A supportive, understanding environment, free of guilt and accusation, is an important factor in recovery. When regrowth of hair is slow or incomplete, both the affected person and the people close to him or her must learn to accept the problem. Alopecia areata is a disorder of hair growth; it should never become a crippling illness.

110

OTHER CAUSES OF HAIR LOSS

Numerous inflammatory processes, drugs, and infections occasionally cause hair loss. In some cases the scalp itself is involved, and the hairless areas are red, tender, or otherwise abnormal. Evaluation by a physician is essential for correct diagnosis and optimum therapy. However, two possibilities are worth considering before seeking professional help.

Severe dandruff can cause enough inflammation to produce diffuse hair loss. Chapter 15 suggests several treatments to improve this condition. If hair thinning is due to dandruff, the hair will return to normal within three months of proper scalp care.

Severe illnesses or changes in hormone balance may cause a dramatic temporary loss of hair, called *telogen effluvium*. A good example of this condition is the hair loss that some women experience one or two months after childbirth, a time of major hormonal adjustment. Discontinuing the use of birth control pills, which simulate pregnancy, may have the same effect. Hair loss occurs in these settings because nearly all the scalp hairs simultaneously enter a resting cycle and then fall out. Normally, not more than one in ten hairs are in the resting or telogen stage, capable of falling out, and hair loss is inconspicuous. Telogen effluvium lasts only a few months before new hairs grow in and the normal proportion between resting and growing hairs is restored. No treatment exists, and indeed none is necessary.

17
Excess Hair

Abundant body hair can be an embarrassing cosmetic problem and may, in some cases, indicate an underlying medical problem.

The amount and distribution of hair is determined by the sex hormones and by hereditary factors (see Chapter 5). The range of "normal" is very wide. Only the palms, soles, and lips are always completely free of hair. *Hirsutism*, the medical term for abundant body and facial hair, is especially common among Caucasians of Southern European ancestry. Men may have prominent hair over the entire trunk and limbs. Women normally have less body and facial hair than men with the same genetic background. However, many completely normal women are more hirsute than many completely normal men. An Italian woman, for example, may have several dark hairs on the chin, around the nipples, and between the navel and pubic area, as well as thick hair on the arms and legs. A man of Asiatic background may have only a scant beard and sparse hair in the underarm and pubic areas. Yet both have normal hormone function.

Hair patterns are usually established during adolescence and generally follow normal, individual courses. Assurance of normality, however, is a small consolation to people who feel the hair is unsightly. There are many ways to get rid of the excess hair, according to a person's preference. It may be removed by shaving or by depilatories, chemicals that dissolve hair. Stray hairs may be plucked with tweezers. None of these processes increases the rate or amount of subsequent hair growth. Dark hairs can be bleached with hydrogen peroxide or, less dramatically, with a weak acid such as lemon juice. A small number of especially bothersome hairs can be permanently removed by electrolysis. In this procedure, a small needle is inserted into the hair follicle and an electric current destroys the hair root. It is best done by a trained electrologist, since pitted scars can result from excess current. Electrolysis is impractical for large areas.

If hirsutism first appears after early adulthood, especially if it occurs over a short period of time, there may be some internal disorder that is treatable. In this case, you should get in touch with your physician.

In the treatment of "normal" excess hair there is no role for sex hormones or indeed for any medications. Do not be misled.

18
Nail
Problems

Problems with fingernails and toenails are very common. Chapter 5 describes the complex process that results in healthy nails — it is easy to see that many things can go wrong. Here we will discuss the most frequent alterations in nail growth and appearance.

Many people complain that they have brittle nails. The nails crack, split, and chip frequently. It is difficult to separate "normal" from "abnormal" in this case. All nails will break if they are bent forcibly enough, often enough. The longer the nails, the more they are subject to repeated trauma. Many people have a habit of tapping their nails against hard surfaces or bending and "testing" them with opposing fingers. Such mechanical stress eventually produces damage. With age, the nail plate normally becomes thinner and more susceptible to injury, so people in their middle years may notice that the nails break more easily than they did in the past.

Rarely, unsuspected disease or nutritional deficiency may cause brittle nails. Any serious, prolonged illness may result in nails that are thin and easily damaged, but in such a situation brittle nails are usually the person's last concern. Similarly, while starvation with severe lack of protein or iron can cause weak nails, a host of other symptoms precedes the nail changes. Thus, a person who is on a diet to lose twenty pounds does not have brittle nails because of nutritional deficiency. There is no validity to the popular myth that eating gelatin or extra protein will strengthen your nails. If your diet already contains adequate protein, as is true for virtually all Americans, your body stores extra food value as fat, not fingernails. If your nails are brittle, the best approach is to keep them fairly short and take care to avoid mechanical injuries, including those you may unwittingly produce yourself. The same applies to slow-growing nails. There is a wide range of normal growth rates at all ages, and in elderly people, nail growth on the feet may almost cease. This is not necessarily a sign of disease and very rarely is it a clue to unrecognized illness. It is annoying if you are waiting for an injured area to "grow out," but such nails are, in fact, a convenience in most cases. Like brittle nails, slow-growing nails may reflect the general body metabolism. Except for maintaining good general health, there is little you can do to improve the situation.

Many people have ridged nails. Grooves or ridges are present in some nails at birth or may develop after a crush injury or other accident. Nearly everyone develops progressive nail ridging with age. Longitudinal ridges, running from the cuticle to the free edge of the nail, are most common and tend to be permanent. Nail ridges begin to appear in many people during early adulthood and have no significance. You cannot prevent them.

Horizontal ridges, running from side to side of the nail, usually represent a specific traumatic event in the life of the nail. Such ridges first appear at the cuticle and grow out with the nail. Single horizontal depressions in each nail plate are called *Beau's lines* and classically indicate a period of acute illness, a brief time when the body made the nail thinner than usual. Since it takes approximately three months for a fingernail to grow the length of the nail bed, if Beau's lines run across the middle of each fingernail, you can guess that an illness or other major stress occurred about six weeks previously.

Nails with many ridges are far more common than those with Beau's lines, however. This type of rippled nail has several causes and is often correctable. If you manicure the nails too vigorously, you may damage the nail base sufficiently to cause a ridge or depression. Habitual misuse of an orange stick, for example, can cause abnormal nail growth. Eczema, psoriasis, or other inflammation in the skin around the nail base can do the same. Most such skin diseases can be controlled with medication, and the nails will then resume normal growth.

A special case of this type is *monilial paronychia*, an infection around the nail bed caused by yeast. The infection tends to be mild and chronic and to affect several fingers. The skin at the nail base is slightly red and swollen; in rare instances a small amount of pus may drain from the cuticle. The nail base may be tender, but often the nail changes are more objectionable than the skin changes. This condition takes many weeks to cure. Your doctor can prescribe medication to apply to the nail base, but it is equally important to keep the fingers dry, since yeast thrive on moisture. This is essential but difficult because many people have paronychia precisely because their jobs or hobbies require putting the hands in water.

In addition to ridges, nails may have spots, stripes, or pits (small craterlike defects); they may "lift up" at the free edge, accumulate crumbly debris under the

116

nail plate, turn color, or become very thick. Such changes sometimes follow injury to a nail. In such cases, usually the cause is obvious and the problem disappears when the nail grows out, in weeks to months. Often, however, such changes are markers of skin disease or fungus infection.

Nail changes accompany many skin diseases, even if the skin near the nails is normal, and may be the only sign of disease. Psoriasis is the best example of this: it may cause any of the abnormalities just mentioned. Yellow-tan discolorations in the nail, called "oil spots," strongly suggest psoriasis even if the person has no skin lesions. The nail changes associated with skin diseases such as psoriasis are rarely permanent and frequently respond to treatment (see Chapter 24).

Fungus often infects toenails and may also infect fingernails. Usually the feet have been involved for years with fine scaling on the soles or moist, split skin between the toes. *Onychomycosis* or fungal infection of nails tends to spread slowly from nail to nail and virtually never clears up without treatment (see Chapter 38).

Ingrown toenails are a common and avoidable problem. Normally, nails are not flat but curve slightly across the toe and enter the skin folds on either side at a gentle angle. An ingrown nail bends too sharply at its edge and enters the skin fold "head on." When the nail is pressed down, its edges push into the skin like dull knives. In time, the skin becomes red and swollen in response to this repeated injury. Ingrown nails are often caused by tight shoes transversely compressing the ends of the toes inside the shoe. This gradually deforms the nail plate, increasing its curvature, so that it occupies a narrower space. As the nail plate bows, its edges become more nearly perpendicular to the skin

117

surface. Then the trouble begins. Early, mild cases can be corrected simply by avoiding ill-fitting shoes. If the nail is ingrown all the way to its cut edge, gently free the embedded corners and round the edge with a nail file, then allow the nails to grow out beyond the tip of the toe. If the toe remains painful despite these steps, consult a podiatrist or dermatologist.

When should you see a doctor because of nail problems? In the case of brittle or slow-growing nails, it is unlikely that your doctor can offer more than reassurance. Rarely, you may have additional subtle signs or symptoms that will prompt your doctor to suspect an underlying condition, such as thyroid disease, which is treatable. In general, if you are otherwise well, you don't need to see a doctor for these problems. If you do not feel well, however, seek a general examination and ask about your nails then.

If you have any of the other nail problems mentioned above, you are quite justified in consulting a dermatologist for diagnosis and treatment (see Chapter 42). Nail conditions are seldom a threat to your health, however, and so the decision to seek medical care should be based on your degree of concern about appearance or possible associated conditions. If your nails are so altered that they cause discomfort or interfere with using your hands or feet, you will definitely benefit from seeing a dermatologist or other trained professional. Such nails can always be improved, if not cured.

A final word: nothing applied to the nails themselves can correct a disease process. The nails are dead, and nail changes only reflect past disturbances in the living cells that made them. Nail polish can hide and therefore solve many nail problems, but bogus treatments only waste time, effort, and money.

118

19

Prominent Blood Vessels

In normal skin blood vessels are invisible. Only the larger veins in the subcutaneous tissue can be seen, most often on the arms and hands as faint blue cords below the skin. However, many people as they age, especially those with a fair complexion, develop fine red lines on the cheeks, nose, and other areas. The medical term for these lines, which are enlarged capillaries and small arteries, is *telangiectasia*. Telangiectasia is often due to chronic excess sun exposure. Over the years the sun damages the blood vessels near the skin surface just as it damages other parts of the skin. Such telangiectasia is permanent. A dermatologist can erase individual blood vessels with a small electric needle when you are in the office, but this procedure is tedious, uncomfortable, and does not always work.

Rosacea is another common cause of facial telangiectasia. This condition resembles acne but begins in middle age rather than in adolescence and produces dilated blood vessels in addition to pimples. The flush and telangiectasia of rosacea are made worse by drinking alcohol or hot beverages such as coffee, by extremes of temperature, and by emotional upsets. Both the pimples and the blood vessel changes may respond to treatment with tetracycline, the antibiotic also used in acne.

High levels of female sex hormones associated with pregnancy and some birth control pills may cause scattered clusters of tiny vessels to appear on the body. This type of telangiectasia usually disappears when hormone levels return to normal.

Several rare diseases cause telangiectasia, especially on the hands, but almost always cause many more striking symptoms first. Occasional telangiectasia is so common in normal people that medical evaluation is not necessary unless there are other unexplained health problems.

Prominent Blood Vessels

20
Itching

Itching can be described as a slightly unpleasant sensation of the skin surface that creates a desire to scratch, rub, or otherwise overpower the body's ability to perceive the itch. Many scientists consider itching a mild form of pain, and some evidence suggests that the same nerves can carry either itch or pain messages to the brain. There are numerous theories to explain how an itch sensation arises in the skin and how it is interpreted in the brain. Undoubtedly, different factors are involved in different types of disorders.

Unlike pain, itching rarely seems useful. Burning your fingers on a hot stove causes you to remove your hand immediately before more tissue injury occurs. Chest pain may warn a patient with heart disease to reduce physical activity before a heart attack occurs. It is more difficult to justify the annoyance of mosquito bites or poison ivy, which itch for hours or days when the damage has already been done. Nevertheless, occasional itchiness is the lot of all people, and some individuals are plagued by severe, persistent itching.

Many rashes are accompanied by itching. *Psoriasis* (Chapter 24) is derived from the Greek word for itching, although in fact many psoriatics do not itch. *Eczema* (Chapter 26) is characterized by severe itching, and people with eczema seem to have a heightened perception of itch, whatever its cause. In many skin disorders, the itchiness appears to be caused by the same inflammation that produces the skin lesions themselves. Appropriate treatment for the rash usually mitigates the symptom.

Itching may also occur when the skin appears normal. Sometimes it is due to dryness, a habitual if not normal state of many people's skin. In this case, regular use of a moisturizer and sensible skin care (see Chapter 7) alleviates the problem.

If the skin is not dry, or if proper grooming does not relieve the itch, other possibilities must be considered. Usually there is no explanation. At times itchiness is suggested by something in the conscious or subconscious mind. (Are you itchy, reading this chapter?) In rare instances, a host of frightening disorders can cause itching in normal-appearing skin. These include liver, thyroid, blood, or kidney disease; drug allergies; cancer or lymphoma; parasitic infestations; and (not so frightening) pregnancy. These possibilities should be considered only if the itching is severe, involves the whole body, and persists for weeks. Even in this case you should not expect the worst. First, a doctor can usually diagnose and treat all these conditions. And, for every itchy person with one of these problems, there are dozens who are completely well except for their annoying symptoms.

Most people are not worried about why they itch; they are simply bothered by itching. Certain factors, chiefly anxiety or stress, exacerbate itching regardless of etiology or severity. An itch that is quite tolerable during the routine of the day may seem intolerable while studying for an exam or awaiting news of a sick family member. Emotional tension does not cause itching but certainly aggravates it.

Scratching is another part of the problem of itching, not part of the cure, as many people believe. Chronic rubbing and scratching may enlarge the cutaneous nerves and make them more susceptible to future itch stimuli. Some terribly itchy skin lesions actually disappear if the person can be prevented from scratching.

A third factor is environmental. Most people realize that rough, tight clothing, especially woolens, may aggravate itching, and some people find synthetic materials, enzyme detergents, and fabric softeners somewhat irritating to their skin. Heat is at least as common an offender, however. Hot baths or showers are temporarily soothing to irritated skin but lead to increased itchiness. Also, sweat, dirt, and many other substances may produce mild irritation and hence promote itching when left on the skin surface for prolonged periods.

Another influence on the severity of itching is the mental energy devoted to the task. Many people experience their worst itching while trying to fall asleep. If the mind and body are unoccupied, the least sensation is magnified. Anxiety, whether about problems suppressed during the day or simply about the possible loss of sleep, keeps the vicious circle going.

Certain areas of the body seem to have a special predilection for itching. The area around the anus is the site of *pruritus ani*, a very annoying disorder that occurs more frequently in men than in women. It can be precipitated by the use of certain oral antibiotics or by diarrhea, but often has no recognized cause. The skin appears normal except for evidence of scratching, whereas itching due to a fungus or yeast infection or psoriasis is associated with redness and scaling around

123

the anal opening. Pruritus ani becomes symptomatic most often after a bowel movement, when itching is triggered by wiping with harsh toilet paper, and at night. Repeated scratching thickens the skin around the anus and this thickening — called lichenification — in turn increases itching. The best therapy for pruritus ani is scrupulous hygiene. If possible, the area should be washed in a bidet or bathtub after each bowel movement and then liberally sprinkled with talcum powder, which prevents chafing of opposing skin surfaces. Toilet paper should be avoided: it is not only inefficient but also irritating to injured skin. Tucks® — cotton flannel discs saturated with witch hazel — are an excellent substitute. Such a regimen controls the problem within a few weeks in most instances. If not, a physician can prescribe a steroid cream to reduce the irritation further, although such creams should be used with caution since they may cause undue thinning of the skin.

Pruritus vulvae is an analogous problem affecting the vulva. Infections due to trichimonas and yeast may also cause itching in this area, but unlike pruritus vulvae they are accompanied by a vaginal discharge. Vulvar itching in postmenopausal women is sometimes due to a lack of estrogen, which can be corrected by daily application of Premarin® cream; but in younger women the cause is unknown and treatment is the same as for pruritus ani. Washing the genital area in a bidet or bathtub after urination and substituting Tucks® for toilet paper are important aspects of therapy. A mild steroid preparation such as hydrocortisone cream may also be necessary initially. As with itching of any etiology, scratching only perpetuates the problem.

124   The best way to manage itching of all types is not to

worry, not to scratch, not to be idle, and not to become overheated. This is in fact sound advice whatever the problems you face, but sometimes difficult or impossible to follow. Other effective treatments for itching include soothing creams, lotions, or sprays for the skin surface and oral medications such as antihistamines or mild tranquilizers. Moisturizers containing menthol or phenol are especially helpful and can be used several times daily. Alcohol-containing preparations cool the skin and may temporarily replace itching with a pleasant tingling sensation, but chronic use can lead to drying and more itching. Cornstarch or a colloidal oatmeal powder (such as Aveeno® or Aveenol®) may be added to a cool or tepid bath once or twice daily for relief. Chlorpheniramine (Chlor-Trimeton®) is a safe, effective antihistamine pill, available without prescription, that may decrease awareness of itching. If these measures are unsuccessful, a physician can select one of a wide range of similar prescription medications for you and adjust the dose according to your body's metabolism and needs. These medicines are especially helpful at bedtime, since all may cause drowsiness as a side effect. Sunbathing sufficient to cause a *slight* sunburn or tan seems to relieve itching of several types and is worth a try, weather permitting.

Topical anesthetics are creams or sprays that temporarily deaden the nerves and hence stop itching. Most end in the letters "caine" or "dryl," and many are sold without prescription. These products are tempting but should be avoided, since allergic reactions may occur and cause a contact dermatitis (Chapter 28). More important, the allergy is permanent and makes it risky to use numerous chemically related drugs, ranging from certain heart medicines to sleeping pills.

Itching is a universal annoyance, usually without

meaning in itself. Simple modifications in behavior can decrease the frequency and severity of itching for many people. Itching associated with skin lesions responds to appropriate medical treatment of the underlying inflammation. Normal-appearing but itchy skin is helped by a variety of creams, lotions, sprays, and bath additives.

When itching is a major problem, your physician can help unravel the complex physiologic and psychologic factors contributing to the condition and can prescribe medication if necessary.

21

Corns

Few of us completely escape these annoying and often quite painful lesions. They occur most commonly on the toes and balls of the feet. Once present, corns seldom disappear, even in young adults. Like calluses, corns are an attempt by the body to protect the affected area from what it perceives as excessive pressure. They are most likely to appear when shoes are ill-fitted or when the bony structure of the foot is abnormal, as in people with hammertoes or some types of arthritis. Many sufferers never notice a problem until the corn appears, however.

The medical term for corn is *clavus*, meaning nail. This aptly describes both the sensation of walking on a corn and its appearance: a firm round area on the surface with a hard waxy pointed core extending about ¼ inch into the skin.

To cure a corn, you must remove the stimulus that produced it. If shoes are too small or pointed at the toe, new, carefully fitted shoes may correct the problem in a matter of months. Shoe bars or space shoes may help, but an orthopedist, podiatrist, or dermatologist should be consulted before you make such an investment. For many people, corrective orthopedic surgery may be necessary for cure. Major surgery to cure a minor discomfort is clearly inappropriate in all but the most extreme cases, especially since very simple and effective treatment is available.

A large number of chemicals and devices are sold, most without prescription, that soften corns and stop the discomfort as long as use is continued, although the corn returns when treatment stops. Dr. Scholl's® various foot pads are a familar example. Salicylic acid plasters — medicated sheets available in most drugstores — offer a second approach. After the daily bath, cut a small pad from the sheet and place it over the corn, then hold it in place with adhesive strip bandages or tape until just before the next bath. Each time the pad is changed, gently remove the softened, dead superficial layers with a pumice stone or other rough surface. When the corn is no longer uncomfortable, apply the plaster for twenty-four hours only every third day or less, as needed, to maintain the improvement. Such home remedies are usually successful, but if pain persists or if you are not completely certain the lesion is a corn, seek professional advice. Your doctor can pare off the tough outer layers of the corn with a surgical blade and prescribe a more potent agent to apply at home.

Corns

22

Skin
Injuries

In its role as protective barrier against the outside world, the skin is often injured. Heat, cold, friction, and pressure all produce damage. Small cuts, scrapes, blisters, and burns are almost daily events. Even without assistance, the skin usually recovers quickly, but often we wish to accelerate this process.

The principal complication of superficial cuts and scrapes is infection. A wound should be rinsed promptly in clean, flowing water. If the surrounding skin is dirty, thorough washing with soap and water is advisable. Brisk bleeding that continues for several minutes causes insignificant blood loss and also removes dirt and germs from the skin. Antibacterial products such as isopropyl (rubbing) alcohol or tincture of iodine may further decrease the number of bacteria in and near the wound. These agents are, however, quite painful on application and seem unnecessarily cruel, especially for children. In addition, chemicals that kill bacteria can also destroy living tissue in the wound and hence delay healing.

After a cut is rinsed, carefully align the skin edges and place an adhesive strip bandage or other dressing across it. If possible, pucker the edges toward each other so that there is no pull on the cut itself. This maneuver speeds healing, minimizes scarring, and helps stop bleeding. Bleeding from an abrasion or scrape can usually be stopped by applying firm pressure through a wad of tissue paper or gauze pad for several minutes. If an attempt to remove this impromptu dressing causes fresh bleeding, leave it in place. If possible, however, cover the nonbleeding surface with an antibacterial ointment such as bacitracin (available without prescription) and then a soft gauze pad. Most of the mismanagement of cuts and scrapes occurs at this point. Dressings on cuts and scrapes are best removed within a day or two — gently, so as not to disrupt healing. Water or hydrogen peroxide helps loosen adherent dressings. If the injury is truly minor, the repair process is already well under way.

Keeping a bandage on the skin provides some protection but unfortunately also provides a warm, moist, dark environment where bacteria thrive. Bacterial counts are more than one-hundredfold higher under a bandage than around an injury exposed to the air. After the first few days a dressing should be used only if the injured area must be exposed to unusually dirty or otherwise inimical surroundings. Even in this situation, the dressing should be loose, so that air can circulate freely underneath.

Puncture wounds, such as those caused by stepping on a nail, usually require a *tetanus booster shot. They should not be treated at home, even if pain and bleeding are minimal.*

Blisters are fluid-filled cavities that may result from virtually any type of skin injury. Unaccustomed manual labor and burns are familiar causes. Usually the epidermis pulls away from the lower layers of skin to

Skin Injuries

form the roof. In time, a new epidermal layer grows across the base of the blister and the now superfluous top layer is shed. When blisters do not prohibit walking, using the hands, or other routine activities, it is best to let them drain and heal at their own rate. Puncturing a blister opens the door to bacteria. Compared with puncturing, complete "deroofing" allows the base to dry, which reduces the risk of infection, but this maneuver also removes the natural protection that the blister roof provided for the thin new skin forming below. The practice of opening blisters with a needle previously "sterilized" in a match flame is particularly unfortunate, since it almost always introduces not only bacteria into the cavity but also small black carbon particles from the flame, which may create a permanent tattoo. If blisters *must* be drained — and this is seldom necessary — use a clean instrument, such as a fresh, individually wrapped razor blade; cut a wide arc in the roof of the blister, holding the blade parallel to the skin surface; gently express the fluid without removing the roof; and apply an antibiotic ointment to the area once or twice daily until healing is complete.

Minor burns rarely blister but may still cause considerable discomfort. Immersing a burned area immediately in cold water reduces the pain considerably and may protect a small margin of skin around the burn from heat damage. A few minutes is sufficient, but no harm is done by keeping the burn cold for a longer period. Do not use ice, since this may superimpose on the burn an injury due to tissue freezing. Frequent applications of a steroid cream, if readily available, may further reduce pain and redness. One application an hour for six hours is usually adequate.

Burns in small children are a special case. Innocent redness following contact with hot water or metal may mask a deep burn. Immersion in cold water is critical, since this has a potentially protective effect. At the first evidence of sloughing or "deep peeling" in such a burn, the child should be examined by a physician experienced in burn injuries. Allowing a moist burn surface to "heal over" by itself may lead to infection and unnecessary scarring.

Because virtually all sunburns are easily avoided (see Chapter 12), it is curious that they are so common. But they are. A moderate to severe sunburn often causes chills, fever, and nausea in addition to painful skin. Once overexposure to sunlight has occurred, there is a grace period of several hours before symptoms appear. During this period or early in the development of redness, a burn reaction may be aborted by high doses of steroid pills, available only by prescription. These pills may cause serious side effects, however, and so can be used only in extreme cases (Chapter 27). They are inappropriate for routine sunburns. For less severe burns, steroid creams may bring some relief, just as they do for thermal burns. Cool baths and soft, loose clothing are helpful. Aspirin, two tablets taken every four hours, may reduce both the burn reaction itself and the accompanying malaise. Products like Solarcaine® and Lanacaine® reduce sunburn discomfort by numbing the skin but cause allergic reactions in some people (Chapter 20). A lotion containing menthol or phenol is nearly as soothing and much less risky. Greasy creams or ointments should be avoided, since they trap heat in the burned skin.

Skin injuries due to cold are much less common than those due to heat but can be equally uncomfortable. Frostbitten skin should be warmed to normal body temperature as quickly as possible, either in warm water or a warm room. Do not heat above 100° F

132

(38° C), since the skin is numb and might be burned without warning pain. Placing frostbitten hands and feet near an open fire or hot radiator is especially dangerous.

In the management of all minor skin injuries three principles should be remembered: cleansing the area, permitting the natural defenses to work, and protecting the area from further damage or contamination. Cleansing includes removing bacteria from the surrounding skin as well as from the wound itself. In order to avoid further injury, the cleansing process should be as gentle as possible. However, wound healing is severely impeded by the presence of any foreign material, and imbedded particles must be removed even if this causes some further tissue injury. Running water from a faucet usually will do the job. Bits of foreign matter not removed in this way can be gently removed with a tweezers sterilized by boiling in water. Within limits, bleeding is beneficial because it helps to cleanse the wound.

Allow a scab to form. The scab represents the body's attempt to restore temporarily the broken physical barrier while waiting for the return of the normal barrier of the healed skin. It is not as effective as intact skin, but protects the cells during healing. Because the scab is more easily damaged than skin, external protection is sometimes helpful, particularly if the wound is in a place likely to be bumped, such as a knee. A loose covering of sterile gauze ordinarily suffices. The bandage should not be airtight, since trapped moisture encourages the growth of bacteria. Plastic adhesive tape is particularly bad in this respect.

If the injury is at a joint where movement is likely to disrupt healing tissues, a splint discourages motion. Pulling the scab loose while changing the dressing retards healing and increases the risk of infection. If the bandage adheres to the scab, hydrogen peroxide or even warm water may be used to loosen it.

The use of topical antiseptics on minor skin injuries is rarely necessary. Any substance that kills bacteria also kills skin and blood cells and thus slows healing. In addition, most bacteria on the skin surface are harmless, and people may be allergic to the antiseptic chemicals. Soap, a relatively ineffective antiseptic, and water remove most bacteria by simply floating them away.

The skin is so well equipped to repair minor damage that any significant interference may slow rather than speed the healing process. When in doubt as to how to manage an injury, do as little as possible. If the injury seems more than trivial, do not hesitate to contact your doctor.

Skin Injuries

23
Acne

Almost everyone has acne at some point. For many, it means an occasional pimple during adolescence; for others, it is a physically and emotionally scarring process that can last twenty years or more.

Acne is caused by obstruction of oil glands that we do not even need. It occurs on the face, back, and chest, where these glands are found. Acne begins when the ducts leading from sebaceous glands to the skin surface become plugged by dead cells, bacteria, and sebum, the oil made in the gland. The first lesion formed is a closed *comedo*, or whitehead. Because the duct is plugged, the normal gland products cannot reach the skin surface and so build up in the skin, making a firm bump. As time passes, the duct wall may stretch as more material accumulates. Finally, the duct opening is quite large. Air can then reach the plug and oxidize its surface. This chemical change plus accumulated pigment darkens the opening. The lesion is then called an *open comedo*, or blackhead. The plug can usually be squeezed out, but the duct may remain enlarged.

As the sebaceous gland continues to function, more

material is forced into the duct. Sometimes the duct wall does not stretch enough and pressure builds up within it. If the wall of the duct is weak, it will rupture, spilling its contents into the skin. Once outside the duct, this material is very irritating to the skin. White blood cells arrive to "clean up." They form a pustule or pimple if the rupture occurred near the skin surface, and a cyst if the rupture occurred deep in the dermis. These lesions are actually small abscesses and may be quite tender. Eventually the inflammation subsides, but if it was severe, a scar forms.

To some extent, the tendency to develop acne is inherited, but some people with severe acne come from families with perfect complexions, and vice versa. Hormonal influences, especially those of the male sex hormone testosterone, are also significant. At puberty, both boys and girls begin to produce testosterone, which activates the oil glands. The glands, which formed before birth but barely functioned in childhood, then enlarge and produce sebum. However, women produce very little testosterone, yet they may have severe acne. Female sex hormones therefore also seem to play a role. Acne in many women is affected by the menstrual cycle and can be exacerbated or improved by birth control pills or pregnancy.

The anatomic structure of the sebaceous glands where acne lesions begin is undoubtedly another factor. Glands with narrow ducts may become plugged more easily than glands with wider ducts. The cellular lining of some sebaceous glands may be more prone to form plugs, regardless of the duct diameter; other ducts may be fragile and rupture easily, producing pimples or cysts. The amount of oil made by the sebaceous glands varies more than tenfold among individuals, and, in general, the greater the oil production, the

136

greater the risk of severe acne. The exact chemical composition of oil and the mechanisms of its breakdown by the ever-present bacteria may also be important. For poorly understood reasons, sleep loss, anxiety, and emotional stresses may aggravate acne. Finally, certain outside influences like oily makeup or prolonged local pressure on the skin play a role in some cases of acne, perhaps by blocking oil ducts.

Acne is *not* caused by chocolate, Coca-Cola®, greasy food, dirt, or masturbation.

Acne is so common that many people, including many physicians, consider it "normal," or at least unworthy of treatment. But acne need not be tolerated or "outgrown." No case of acne is too mild or too severe for therapy. Although incurable, acne can virtually always be improved considerably by current methods of treatment, which reduce both the number of active lesions and the risk of acne scarring.

Proper washing is a cornerstone of acne therapy. The skin should be kept moderately dry, but not red or sore, by regular use of an abrasive soap such as Fostex® or Brasivol®. A cleaning sponge such as a BUF-PUF® may also be used, instead of a washcloth, if tolerated. Such washing removes surface oil, dead skin, and dirt, all of which can occlude pores, and loosens the existing plugs. The increased cell turnover that results from this mechanical stimulation may also help prevent comedo formation. Once a day is usually sufficient. If the skin remains oily despite washing twice daily, change to a more abrasive soap or add an acne gel or lotion (see below). There is no benefit in washing many times each day with regular soap. This eventually causes severe dryness without treating the acne. The same is true of washing with alcohol or astringents.

For very oily skin, there are numerous gels and lotions that help to dry acne lesions. Such products contain sulfur, resorcinol, salicylic acid, or benzoyl peroxide in varying concentrations. Benzoyl peroxide also kills bacteria, which contribute to the inflammation of pimples and cysts, and hence offers an advantage over the other compounds. Several preparations containing benzoyl peroxide such as Benoxyl® and Persadox® are available without prescription. It is worth trying several products, one at a time, to find one well-suited to your skin. Each of these products should be applied once daily, after washing, and left in contact with the skin. If redness or excessive dryness develops, stop for several days, then try alternate-day applications. If oiliness persists, try twice-daily applications or a more concentrated form of the medication.

Exposure to the sun seems to be excellent acne treatment for some people. Those who cover facial lesions with their hair or refuse to wear a bathing suit because of acne cysts may be doing themselves a disservice. Painful burns are not necessary, but frequent sunbathing, as tolerated, sometimes improves acne and the tan at least helps to make the lesions less noticeable. When sun is available, rely on it and reduce the amount of other therapy.

A commercial reflector-type sunlamp, which costs approximately $15, may be used daily during the winter or when sunbathing is otherwise impossible. It is usually not as helpful as natural sunlight but worth trying in some resistant cases. The eyes must be protected and all treatments carefully timed to prevent unnecessary and sometimes serious burns. Give three separate exposures (left, right, and front) with the lamp at a distance of one foot from the face. Begin with twenty seconds per exposure and increase by five or ten seconds daily until mild sunburn results; then increase treatment times very cautiously, perhaps five seconds every three days. If you skip treatments, subtract five seconds from the last dose for each day missed. Daily treatments are much safer and more effective than sporadic ones.

People frequently wonder if it is helpful or harmful to squeeze pimples and blackheads. In general, it is helpful to remove blackheads. A lesion resistant to gentle squeezing may be removed by centering an eyedropper over it, perpendicular to the skin, so that downward pressure forces the blackhead up into the hollow bevel. This prevents inflammation from beginning in the plugged gland and improves the skin's appearance. Blackheads reform after two or three months, however, so an abrasive soap should still be used daily. It is not harmful to open gently and drain superficial pimples, but deep cysts are often made worse. Serious infection or increased scarring can result from manipulating these deep lesions.

Small changes in habits, mannerisms, and grooming can greatly improve acne in some people. *External pressure on acne-prone skin can cause lesions.* For example, soldiers or even hiking enthusiasts sometimes develop severe acne under their backpacks, as do athletes under their protective sports gear. *Leaning the face on one or both hands while poring over a book or during sleep can have the same effect.* Even the unconscious gesture of covering acne lesions when talking to others is detrimental. Altering such habits can lead to dramatic improvement in some cases. Combing the hair over acne on the forehead and cheeks is occlusive, prevents sun exposure, and deposits an oily film on the skin. Virtually all makeups, especially oily "pancake" types, eventually worsen acne for the same reason.

If the steps already listed do not produce a marked improvement within two to three months, consider seeing a dermatologist, who can analyze the factors contributing to your acne, recommend medications not available without a doctor's prescription, and perform delicate procedures to improve deep-seated lesions.

Tetracycline is an antibiotic widely prescribed for acne treatment. Used in conjunction with one of the surface drying agents, it improves pimples and cysts in more than nine out of ten patients. As an antibiotic, it kills bacteria, including those on the skin. Although the bacteria themselves do no harm, they do metabolize sebum into irritating acids that may exacerbate acne lesions. Acne is not a simple bacterial infection, however, and once the antibiotic is stopped, acne returns. To be effective, tetracycline must be continued throughout the acne-prone years, although usually a low dose suffices.

Fortunately, tetracycline is a very safe and inexpensive medication, so prolonged treatment is possible for most people who benefit from it. There are only two common problems. A mild feeling of nausea may occur, especially after large early morning doses, but this can usually be avoided by taking the capsules one at a time or later in the day. (Since milk and food prevent absorption from the stomach, tetracycline must be taken at least thirty minutes before meals, however.) The second problem affects women only. It is a tendency to yeast infections of the vagina (see Chapter 33), especially if birth control pills are being used. A woman prone to yeast infections should mention this to her doctor when tetracycline is prescribed, so steps can be taken to reduce the risk and to allow prompt treatment if symptoms appear. A vinegar douche (one tablespoonful in a pint of tepid water) twice weekly

140

may prevent some yeast infections, and several prescription medicines are even more effective.

A number of other antibiotics also improve acne and can be used if tetracycline fails. Certain antibiotics are helpful when applied directly to skin lesions as creams or lotions, and this form of therapy may eventually replace antibiotic pills and capsules.

Scarring is probably the worst aspect of acne, since it remains for life. Some people are truly disfigured, but often improve with time. For such people, dermabrasion and chemical peels may substantially improve the skin's appearance. However, there is no magic way to remove scars. The techniques now available essentially replace pitted, irregular scars with a larger area of smooth scar that may look very attractive under makeup, but rarely has the appearance or texture of normal skin. The procedures are quite uncomfortable, and many weeks are required for complete healing. Infections, permanent pigment alteration, and prominent scarring are possible, although uncommon, complications. Dermabrasion and chemical peels are not valid treatments for mild acne scarring and should never be performed if new lesions have appeared within the past year. A new technique erases individual scars by the injection of silicone underneath the pitlike depression but is not yet approved for general use. A plastic surgeon can sometimes replace large pits with less visible scars, but this approach is impractical if many lesions are present.

In summary, acne is a common, sometimes severe, but always treatable disease. Proper therapy can greatly reduce the number of lesions and can prevent much of the scarring that occurs in severe cases. And Time, the great healer, eventually tames even the worst acne.

24
Psoriasis

I have long been a potter, a bachelor, and a leper. Leprosy is not exactly what I have, but what in the Bible is called leprosy (see Leviticus 13, Exodus 4:6, Luke 5:12–13) was probably this thing, which has a twisty Greek name it pains me to write. The form of the disease is as follows: spots, plaques, and avalanches of excess skin, manufactured by the dermis through some trifling but persistent error in its metabolic instructions, expand and slowly migrate across the body like lichen on a tombstone. I am silvery, scaly. Puddles of flakes form wherever I rest my flesh. Each morning, I vacuum my bed. My torture is skin deep: there is no pain, not even itching; we lepers live a long time, and are ironically healthy in other respects. Lusty, though we are loathsome to love. Keen-sighted, though we hate to look upon ourselves. The name of the disease, spiritually speaking, is Humiliation.*

The heartbreak of psoriasis is no joke. The truth is, psoriasis is a disfiguring and unpredictable condition that can be emotionally crippling, physically uncomfortable, and in very rare cases, even life-threatening. Psoriasis has been a curse throughout history and is nearly as much of a stigma today as it was in biblical

* From "The Journal of a Leper," a short story by John Updike about a man with psoriasis, which appeared in *The New Yorker*, July 19, 1976. (Reprinted with permission of the author and *The New Yorker*.)

times when psoriatics were grouped with lepers. Treatment, for social as well as medical reasons, is often demoralizing, inconvenient, and expensive. In the United States each year psoriasis costs its four to eight million victims many millions of dollars and thousands of days lost from work. And these are not the only costs. The shame and embarrassment caused by psoriasis are so great that victims refuse to expose their lesions, even if it means forgoing swimming and other activities that call for revealing attire. It is significant that many people have never seen psoriasis, even though almost everyone has an acquaintance who is afflicted.

Involved areas become red, thickened, and scaly because of increased blood flow and a heaping-up of rapidly multiplying, not quite mature, epidermal cells. This hectic metabolism may persist in a patch of skin for many years or may suddenly revert to normal. It is always potentially reversible. Certain areas, such as the elbows, knees, and scalp are most commonly affected, but in rare cases the entire skin surface may become involved. Psoriasis tends to appear in injured areas of skin, such as those of a scratch or burn, as the skin heals. Psoriasis affects only the skin and nails; other body tissues are normal.

The tendency for psoriasis is inherited. In families with a history of psoriasis, about one person in seven has psoriatic skin lesions, compared to 2 to 4 percent of the general population. People who develop psoriasis are born with the tendency, even though the skin lesions may first appear at any time from infancy to old age. Nevertheless, many psoriatics are the only family members affected. You are not a potential victim of psoriasis just because a relative has the disease. You must inherit several distinct genetic messages. This   *143* often does not happen, even if all the necessary genes are in the family's genetic pool. Nor does it mean you must develop psoriasis if you have all the responsible genes. In some cases only one of two identical twins who have exactly the same genes ever develops psoriasis.

Psoriasis is not contagious. You cannot get it from or give it to another person.

The course of psoriasis is unpredictable. Psoriasis may begin at any time in life, from infancy to old age. It may remain confined to a few small areas, or spread, or even progress to involve the entire skin surface. Psoriasis may disappear completely for many years, but more often it waxes and wanes around its established norm. There is no way for a psoriatic or a physician to predict how extensive or troublesome the condition will be.

Certain factors do aggravate psoriasis in many people, however. Emotional stresses, such as problems at home or work or a death in the family, frequently produce a flare-up in people with stable psoriasis. Heavy drinking is often associated with more severe psoriasis, perhaps because of underlying stresses. The same relationship seems to hold for obesity. Another common aggravating factor is habitual rubbing, picking, or scratching of affected areas such as the groin, shins, and scalp. Such repeated trauma actually provokes the skin to produce more epidermal cells, negating treatment intended to reduce cell proliferation. Certain bacterial infections, especially a "strep throat," can produce sudden, widespread psoriatic involvement in predisposed people.

The appearance of the lesions is the major problem, but psoriasis may also itch at times and, especially on the palms and soles, may cause painful cracks. Severe

144

nail involvement can produce mechanical as well as cosmetic problems if the nails "catch" frequently. In rare instances, psoriasis is so extensive that the extra blood flow to the skin creates a strain on the heart or prevents proper regulation of body temperature. All these problems can be corrected by appropriate treatment of the psoriasis itself.

There is one problem associated with psoriasis that is not related to the severity of the skin lesions. This is arthritis. The great majority of psoriatics are spared, but about 5 percent develop a characteristic inflammation of one or more joints, often affecting the fingers. It may be mild or crippling, much more or much less of a problem than the skin lesions. Psoriatic arthritis should be cared for by a physician with specific knowledge of this problem, since new medical and surgical treatments are constantly being made available.

There is no cure for psoriasis, but there are many effective treatments. Each approach to therapy has advantages and disadvantages; each individual responds in his or her own way. At best, psoriasis is a significant, recurring, and disheartening problem. For all these reasons, the key to successful treatment of psoriasis is often a lasting relationship with a physician who is knowledgeable about the disease. Usually this is a dermatologist. Certainly no one should be resigned to a life of untreated psoriasis before consulting such an expert. The treatment modalities discussed below are usually less effective — and often unobtainable — without your physician's advice and consent.

Sun exposure is often an excellent treatment for psoriasis. People with mild psoriasis may clear completely if they are able to sunbathe regularly. It is not necessary to get sunburned, and indeed a sunburn can make psoriasis much worse. Children's lesions may disappear during summer vacation; harried working adults may benefit inside and out from a two-week Caribbean vacation. Many dermatologists believe that the face is spared in most patients with psoriasis largely because it receives the greatest year-round sun exposure.

The tremendous potential benefit of sunshine often cannot be realized, however. Many people are unwilling to expose their skin lesions in public and in any case cannot expose the genitalia and breasts. People must often work during the midday hours, when the sun is strongest, and the weather is frequently forbidding. These obstacles can be surmounted by using artificial ultraviolet light. A standard sunlamp is impractical because it can treat only one small area at a time, but commercially available four-foot fluorescent tubes may be aligned on a board so that two exposures (front and back) treat the entire skin surface. Such a home treatment device is convenient and permits optimal, daily exposures, *but can be exceedingly dangerous.* It should be constructed by an electrician (expected cost, $500–$1,000) and must be used only with goggles to protect the eyes and a timing device to avoid burns from overexposure. A much better solution for most people is to use a "light box," a cabinet lined with artificial ultraviolet bulbs, in their dermatologist's office or hospital clinic, usually three times weekly until the skin lesions clear. Psoriasis is one situation in which the benefits of ultraviolet light often outweigh the risks (see Chapters 12 and 13).

Tar and related products are helpful in psoriasis, and most are available without prescription. Refined tar may be added to the bath or applied directly to skin lesions overnight as a cream, gel, or paste. Regular use of a tar-containing shampoo can often control even severe scaling on the scalp. Until the 1950s, tar was central to psoriasis treatment and is still used frequently in conjunction with ultraviolet therapy for hospitalized patients. It is safe and relatively inexpensive. The only problem is the mess. In general, tar products look and smell like tar. They may stain skin, hair, nails, clothes, and everything else. Fortunately, a much less offensive tar gel, Estar®, has recently been developed and may herald a new generation of these useful compounds.

A number of products called *keratolytics* remove thick adherent scales from psoriatic lesions. They may be creams, pastes, or gels and usually contain salicylic acid and other irritating chemical agents. A keratolytic agent is most effective when applied to moistened skin or scalp, covered with plastic (gloves, shower cap, or a sheet of plastic wrap) and left in place four to eight hours. Applications should be repeated daily until the scales are gone. Sometimes this step is necessary before sunlight or medication can penetrate the involved skin.

Corticosteroids are very potent hormones, normally made in small amounts by the adrenal glands, that revolutionized the treatment of psoriasis and many other skin diseases in the 1950s when they were first synthesized in the laboratory. Today, dozens of steroid compounds are available for topical use. Steroids for psoriasis are usually applied to the affected skin two or three times daily as a vanishing cream, ointment, or lotion. The specific steroid preparation prescribed for your skin depends on the area to be treated, the severity of the lesions, your response to previous medications, and several other factors. Like keratolytics, steroids are more effective when used under plastic wrap, but your physician must advise you on whether to use this technique on a given lesion, since skin can

147

be damaged by overuse of these potent medications. When used as prescribed, steroids can safely flatten and often eradicate lesions, but proper use is expensive and tedious. Steroid preparations are less messy than tar but nearly as difficult to apply and must be used faithfully for weeks or months for best results. Occasionally a doctor may choose to inject steroids into a stubborn spot, but this technique should not be overused. Steroid pills and intramuscular injections have been largely abandoned by conscientious physicians despite their appeal for patients, because the medication often causes severe side effects when used in this way and because psoriasis may flare up so badly that hospitalization is required if the pills or shots are stopped.

Usually, mild to moderate psoriasis can be well controlled by some combination of these treatments. Once a successful program is found, your physician needs to see you only once or twice a year unless problems arise. Psoriatic lesions should be minimal or absent most of the time.

Severe psoriasis involves somewhat different expectations and treatment programs. By definition, psoriasis is severe when it is extensive and does not clear in a reasonable time period with ultraviolet light, tar, keratolytic agents, and steroids. *Antimetabolites* are often prescribed for people with severe psoriasis who are otherwise in good health. Originally, such drugs were developed to treat cancer and are still used in this way. They interfere with cell division and so prevent the rapid epidermal growth of psoriasis. Unfortunately, they also poison cells in the liver, bone marrow, stomach and intestinal walls, and many other organs. Hence, the dose must be carefully calculated to improve the psoriasis without damaging normal tissue.

Because they impede normal development, antimetabolites should almost never be used by growing children and absolutely never by people who are attempting to conceive a child, since gametes (eggs or sperm) in either prospective parent could form abnormally, and a developing fetus would be deformed by the drug in the mother's bloodstream. Despite all these potential problems, certain antimetabolites have proven remarkably safe and effective in carefully selected, carefully monitored patients. Methotrexate is prescribed most often, usually as pills taken in divided weekly doses. The medication must be continued for many months, and psoriatic lesions usually return soon after it is stopped. Aside from the need for frequent blood tests, antimetabolites are convenient and popular among patients who have not experienced complications.

Periodic hospitalization is sometimes necessary to control severe psoriasis and may produce a complete remission for months or even years. Effective hospitalization usually calls for specially trained nurses and physicians as well as facilities such as an ultraviolet light box. The complicated 24-hours-a-day regimen of topical skin treatments, baths, shampoos, and light exposures exceeds the capabilities of most community hospitals, even though psoriatics are usually in better general health than the other patients. This discrepancy between basically healthy patients and the need for sophisticated treatment has led in recent years to the creation of several psoriasis day-care centers. Patients arrive in the morning and receive intensive treatment all day, but return home at night. The cost is much less than for the same care in a general hospital, and most people prefer the ambience. In either a hospital or a special day-care center, usually two to four weeks of continuous therapy is necessary to clear psoriasis.

A new option for treating severe psoriasis is the combined use of psoralen (see Chapter 14), a photoactive drug, and long-wave ultraviolet light, called UV-A. This therapy is known as PUVA. Like methotrexate, psoralen is taken by mouth and reaches all body tissues, but psoralen differs in that it affects cells only in the presence of ultraviolet energy. Since these wavelengths do not penetrate beyond the skin, psoriasis can be controlled without risk to internal organs. The patient takes the pills at home or work, comes to the doctor's office or clinic two hours later, disrobes, and stands in a specially designed ultraviolet treatment cabinet for approximately ten to thirty minutes twice a week. In about nine out of ten patients, the psoriasis gradually disappears over two to three months. Time lost from other activities amounts to one or two hours per week, rather than hours each day with conventional therapy.

Psoriasis is analogous in many ways to diabetes mellitus (sugar diabetes): both are common, chronic, inherited diseases. Most of the symptoms of diabetes can be well controlled by daily injections of the hormone insulin or by careful regulation of the diet or by both. These treatments for diabetes do not cure the disease, however; once acquired it lasts a lifetime. Similarly, treatment for psoriasis does not cure the disease but only suppresses the skin lesions. Often treatment may be stopped temporarily in either diabetes or psoriasis, but flare-ups occur unless treatment is resumed periodically or a maintenance program is instituted. Just as diabetes can be mild or severe, psoriasis may result in only a few occasional patches or be extremely widespread; it may be easy to manage or virtually resistant to standard treatments, requiring hospitalization for control.

Psoriasis is at best a nuisance and at worst a living nightmare. It cannot be cured. If it goes away, it almost always comes back. Treatment is difficult or dangerous or both. However, the plight of a person with psoriasis can be ameliorated by family, friends, and physician. Psoriatics need encouragement, not criticism. If those close to them are optimistic and supportive, most people with psoriasis are able to deal effectively with the problems. Moreover, in order to benefit from this help, a psoriatic must be honest about the disease and the disappointments and frustrations it may engender. A strong, open relationship between psoriatics and their intimate associates is critical to successful treatment.

25
Warts

Warts are one of the most common infections of man. They are caused by a specific virus that can enter the skin through small scrapes or cuts, multiply in the living cells of the epidermis, and induce the skin to overgrow, forming characteristic rough bumps. The wart virus infects only the upper layers of the epidermis; hence, a wart is a very superficial infection. Warts do not have "roots" and never involve the deeper layers of skin. And contrary to persistent popular belief, they cannot be acquired from handling frogs or from other socially disparaged behavior.

Plantar warts are so named because they are on the plantar surface of the foot (the sole). They are often incorrectly called "planter's warts" and believed to be more serious or somehow different from other warts. They may be painful, unlike warts in most locations, because they are on a weight-bearing surface, but they are just plain warts. Sexually transmitted warts, also called *condyloma accuminata*, occur on the genitalia and may be caused by a slightly different virus. These are discussed in Chapter 37.

Warts are unlike most common virus infections

(such as measles, chicken pox, and German measles) in that many people are never affected while others are plagued for years. We now know that people who get warts have a specific susceptibility, a "blind spot" in their immune defense systems. Therefore, although warts are contagious, whether you develop them or not depends more on your inborn ability to fight the infection than on how often you are exposed to the virus. Quarantine makes sense for smallpox and mumps but not for warts. Unfortunately, our society is still afraid of "spreading" warts. Many public swimming pools and camps refuse to permit youngsters with warts to use their facilities. This attitude toward warts is unjustified and puts quite a burden on affected families.

Warts are harmless, but may be uncomfortable, especially on the sole of the foot, and are often unsightly. What can you do about them?

One valid alternative is to do nothing. Nine out of ten warts go away by themselves, untreated, within two years. While it is true that warts may spread from one spot to another on the skin, the removal of all the existing warts will not necessarily prevent new ones from appearing. Again, with this virus, it seems to be a matter of susceptibility, not availability.

Anything that destroys the virus-infected epidermal cells of a wart will cure it. The problem in treating a wart is one of adjusting the severity of the treatment to the severity of the disease. Clearly, you don't amputate a leg because of warts on the foot. In general, it is best to begin with something mild that kills a few cells, hopefully enough to cure the wart, and that doesn't leave a scar. Anyone or any product label guaranteeing to cure every wart without leaving a scar is misleading you.

153

Warts

An all too frequent practice among desperate wart victims of all ages is to attempt to bite or cut the lesions off. In theory, this can work, but it usually doesn't. Moreover, it invites infection and brisk bleeding and may spread the warts to other areas, such as the lips. Other remedies are more sanitary and more effective.

Several chemicals, such as Compound W®, are available without prescription and are often worth trying. To be safe and effective, they must be used regularly, according to directions. Plan on at least a month of daily treatment for most warts. This approach is relatively inexpensive and painless.

Many people seek professional help either because the drugstore remedies have failed or because they desire a faster cure. In general, podiatrists (for plantar warts) and dermatologists (for all warts) have the broadest experience and the best equipment. For many warts, the doctor will choose cryotherapy (freezing) with liquid nitrogen. This substance has a temperature of $-196°$ C and easily kills epidermal cells when applied to the surface of a wart. One treatment is often sufficient for small warts; if warts are very large or numerous, several treatments, usually at one-to-three-week intervals, are necessary. Anesthesia is not needed, but the wart area throbs and "burns" during the fifteen-to-thirty-second freezing period and may be sensitive for several days afterward. This procedure almost never causes a scar but, like most treatments, cures only about 60 percent of warts during the first visit.

Electrodesiccation, destruction of warts with electric current, is another common and useful treatment, but has a slightly higher risk of scarring than does liquid nitrogen therapy. A number of strong acids and other

154

tissue-destroying chemicals can be applied to warts by an experienced professional, with comparably good results after several visits.

In the case of plantar warts, surgical removal is still common. Occasionally warts are so bothersome and resistant to other treatment that excision is warranted. However, always remember that eventually most warts disappear without treatment and that all surgical procedures leave scars. On the sole of the foot, scars may be painful, just like the warts they replace. And unlike warts, scars are permanent.

An increasingly popular technique for plantar warts is blunt dissection. This is similar to surgical excision but uses a scooplike device instead of a knife. As in conventional surgery, local anesthesia is used. When sensation returns a few hours later, there is enough discomfort to limit walking for a day or two but less than after most wart treatments. The cure rate is high, about 80 percent, and blunt dissection rarely leaves a scar. If you are considering surgical removal of a wart, ask your doctor or podiatrist about this technique.

Then there is hypnotism. Self-hypnotism seems to be the basis of such folk-medicine cures as throwing a potato over the roof. Formal hypnotic suggestion by a psychiatrist or other trained physician can eradicate warts in at least some individuals, although the reason for these cures is completely unknown. Children under ten years of age are especially receptive to hypnosis, but certain adults are also good candidates. This approach has the great advantage of being painless and easy for the patient and is especially practical for treating warts in young children. Unfortunately, the response of warts to this treatment is not especially reliable. Some warts do not improve at all. The possible

155

beneficial influence of "suggestion" can always be added to more conventional treatments, however. A child who is convinced by parents or physician that a certain medication will remove warts may actually have a better chance for cure than a skeptical sibling.

Recurrent warts in shaved skin are a special case. They appear most often in men's beard areas but may also affect women's legs, for example. The razor cuts through warts, exposing living virus to the skin surface and then transmits the virus into minute nicks and scrapes in other areas. Weeks to months later, the new warts become apparent, and the cycle continues. Such warts should be treated promptly by one of the approaches mentioned above. In addition, shaving habits must change temporarily. For at least a few months, stop shaving or use a depilatory to avoid cutting the skin surface.

Warts are so commonplace that most people feel comfortable with self-diagnosis. If you think you have a wart, you are probably right. However, some malignant tumors and other significant lesions may be mistaken for warts. If a "wart" grows rapidly, bleeds easily, first appears after age forty, or seems unusual, it should be checked by a physician.

Warts are a harmless but unpopular virus infection. There are many effective treatments, but these are often slow or incomplete if scarring is to be avoided. Don't expect miracles of your druggist or your physician and take solace in the fact that most warts eventually disappear, with or without treatment.

Warts

26

Eczema

Eczema has been called "the itch that rashes." The word is derived from a Greek term for "bubbling over," a good description for the way lesions begin, as small blisters or bubbles in previously normal skin. Dermatologists sometimes designate as eczema any rash with this appearance, regardless of its cause. For most people, however, eczema refers to a rather specific skin disease — itchy, thickened patches that wax and wane for years, often affecting people who also have allergies, asthma, or hay fever. For the purpose of this chapter, eczema is this very common and chronic condition, sometimes also referred to as *atopic dermatitis* or *atopic eczema*. Hand eczema and primary irritant dermatitis are discussed in Chapter 28.

The cause of eczema is unknown. A tendency to develop eczema is inherited and seems to be, to a certain extent, the result of a "hypersensitivity" to the environment, although eczema is not an allergy. Not all children in a family with eczema inherit the disorder. Statistically, most do not. Indeed, only about 70 percent of people with eczema are aware of *any* affected relatives.

Dry skin, an increased number of creases on the palms, and a prominent skin fold in the lower eyelids (*Dennie's lines*) are often present at birth in people destined to have eczema. Blood vessels in the skins of these people constrict readily. A firm stroke with an object such as a pen cap can produce a pale line that lasts several minutes before blood flow returns to normal, while in people without eczema such a stroke stimulates blood vessels to dilate and causes a red mark on the skin. Also common among people with eczema are cold hands and feet, possibly because of constricted blood vessels and decreased blood flow in these areas. The fact that these minor abnormalities involve the entire skin surface and persist throughout life, whether or not skin lesions are present, suggests that the basic skin structure of people with eczema may be subtly different from the normal.

The most obvious abnormality of eczema skin cannot be seen. It is a striking tendency to itch. Warmth, contact with soap or rough clothing, and emotional tension may provoke intolerable bouts of itching. Itching leads to scratching. Scratching and rubbing produce the skin lesions of eczema. Without scratching, the skin may continue to itch but appears completely normal. It cannot be overemphasized that rubbing and scratching the skin perpetuate eczema.

Although the tendency is inborn, eczema is very rare at birth. It begins most commonly in childhood, but sometimes later, and may last for a few weeks or a lifetime. There may be a single small patch of eczema or the entire skin surface may be red, weepy, scaly, and itchy. Eczema is quite unpredictable, but there are some patterns. Of all children with eczema, about one in three is still bothered by rashes twenty years later. If the child also has asthma or a strong family background of eczema, allergies, and asthma, the chance of persistent eczema is greater. Mild eczema usually remains mild. Some cases of severe childhood eczema disappear completely after a few years but are more likely to flare periodically for decades. Of all people with eczema, about half eventually develop asthma, allergies, or hay fever.

The location of eczema of the body often changes with age. In the first year of life, eczema tends to affect the face and scalp most severely. Over the next several years, lesions shift away from the face to the trunk. By adolescence, usually the flexures of the elbows and knees are the principal sites. Eczema is not "spread" by scratching as an infection may be, but rather follows its own internal rhythm.

Eczema often invites other medical problems. Blistered lesions and especially scratch marks are an open door for bacteria wishing to infect the skin. Impetigo (Chapter 30) and occasionally deeper infections result. If not treated promptly, these bacterial infections may lead to scarring on the skin or to several internal illnesses.

Certain viruses spread easily on the skin of people with eczema. A smallpox vaccination (live attenuated vaccinia virus) may produce a severe, widespread, and even fatal eruption, very similar to the disease it is intended to prevent. A cold sore (*herpes simplex*) may behave in the same way (see Chapter 31). This complication may occur whether or not eczema is present at that moment. The susceptibility to severe infection is not a simple matter of breaks in the skin barrier. For this reason, no one with eczema or a history of eczema should ever be vaccinated except under extraordinary circumstances. School and immigration authorities respect this precaution and waive vaccination requirements for people with appropriate letters from their physicians. Individuals with eczema should also avoid contact with recently vaccinated people and those with active cold sores.

People with eczema may be prone to certain allergies, both *contact dermatitis* (see Chapter 28) and drug reactions. Penicillin, a frequent allergen in general, should be avoided if possible.

The emotional and social ramifications of eczema dwarf the medical problems. Consider the plight of a baby with eczema. An itchy baby cries, fusses, tears at its skin, and makes extra demands on its parents. Its appearance and behavior provoke parental guilt and anger. The normal physical intimacy between mother and child is disturbed by the disease and its treatment. Stroking, bathing, and dressing do not produce pleasant sensations in the baby's skin. Instead, these early human contacts result in itching and burning. As the child grows older, it learns to be ashamed of its skin lesions. This attitude begins a vicious circle of eczema, emotional tension, more eczema. The victim's self-image is distorted. Eczema sufferers learn to manipulate their parents and other adults by scratching and exacerbating the skin lesions. In so doing, they sometimes lose their best allies in the struggle against eczema. It is not surprising that people with eczema are sometimes characterized as tense and resentful.

Eczema cannot be cured, but affected individuals, their families, and their physicians can do much to improve the condition. Perhaps the most important safeguard is to avoid stimuli that provoke itching.

Very hot, cold, or dry environments or rapid temperature changes may induce itching. Sweat makes itching worse. A person with eczema should live in a climate that is warm and damp year-round. In less than ideal climates, accommodations must be made. Rooms should be kept at 68° to 70° F. A cool-mist humidifier should be used at least in the bedroom during the dry winter months in northern climates and all year in arid ones. Such a humidifier is not noisy or steamy and costs as little as $30. Clothing is important. Wool, silk, rough fabrics, and tightly fitting garments cause trouble. Parents may unintentionally aggravate a child's eczema by overdressing him or her in cold weather or by not promptly removing coats and sweaters when the child is in the house. Intense physical exercise raises body temperature rapidly and may cause itching. Strenuous sports are best avoided by children and young adults with bad eczema. Very hot or spicy foods may also cause itching.

Anything that moisturizes the skin is beneficial: bath oils, emollient creams such as Eucerin®, or even vegetable shortening. A moisturizer should be applied after every bath and whenever the skin feels dry.

Chapter 7 discusses problems arising from excess bathing and soap.

Fatigue may increase itching. A person with eczema should cultivate regular sleep patterns. Stress is notorious for making eczema worse. Some stresses are difficult to avoid; they are inherent in family life, jobs, and school. Whenever possible, however, mental and emotional stress should be circumvented: cramming for exams, driving at rush hour, forcing unwanted music lessons on the children, Christmas shopping on December 24. A sense of humor is always helpful. Sympathetic understanding from family, friends, teachers, or employers is invaluable.

A person with moderate or severe eczema needs medical attention. Prescription drugs to relieve itching and inflammation plus prompt treatment of complications reduce eczema from a nightmare to a manageable problem.

Steroid creams and ointments are the mainstay of eczema therapy. They reduce both itching and inflammation. The dozens of steroid preparations available allow the physician to choose one well suited to your skin lesions. In general, a cream is best if lesions are weepy or tend to become infected, because creams are drying. An ointment keeps the skin more moist and is usually less irritating to scratched skin than a cream; the same amount of steroid medication for the same price is more effective in an ointment than in a cream base. These features make ointments desirable for most eczema. Unfortunately, people with eczema as well as their doctors often sacrifice the greater effectiveness of ointments to the greaseless elegance of creams. It is a poor exchange.

Another regrettable practice is too frequent use of the steroid medication. Six applications are six times as costly and time-consuming as, but less effective than, one application, covered by plastic and left on for two to four hours. Steroids penetrate the skin barrier best when applied immediately after the bath or shower and covered with a nonbreathing plastic sheet. A material such as Saran Wrap® can be used to encircle arms and legs, for example. Such occlusive wraps cannot be used by small children, of course, because of the potential for accidental suffocation. Fortunately, a child's skin is less resistant to steroids than an adult's and almost always responds to treatment without occlusion. Steroids may be overutilized, to be sure. Prolonged regular use, especially with occlusive dressings, can lead to permanent, undesirable skin changes and should be undertaken only with close medical supervision.

Steroid medication in the form of pills or injections often clears eczema dramatically but is almost never worth the risks. These risks are discussed in Chapter 24, Psoriasis, another condition for which this tempting mode of therapy is unwise.

Antihistamine pills for adults or elixir for children both relieve itching and act as mild tranquilizers. Some people need only small doses at bedtime; others need larger doses every four to six hours while awake to suppress itching and scratching. When eczema is severe, regular use of antihistamines for several days may be necessary to break the itch-scratch cycle that creates and perpetuates the skin lesions. Concern about long-term usage of such medication is legitimate, however. It can make people drowsy. It may prevent a child from concentrating at school or endanger an adult operating heavy machinery or driving a car. Nevertheless, uncontrolled symptoms of eczema can be even more devastating and certainly justify liberal use of antihistamines. In certain cases, several days of complete bed-rest with adequate sedation can dramatically improve eczema.

Tar derivatives sooth eczema. They are inexpensive and have fewer potential problems than steroid creams or ointments but are certainly messier. Bath additives are probably the easiest tar products to use. A capful of Balnetar®, Zetar®, or similar emulsion can be added to a warm bath, after the regular bath or shower. The tar bath is for relaxation and treatment of the eczema, not for washing. Allow fifteen or twenty minutes.

Most important, people with eczema need perspective on it. They must not feel that their skin controls their lives. Family, close friends, and a physician — all of whom can provide emotional and medical support — help eczema victims to overcome their problems.

163

27
Poison Ivy

There is a great deal of misinformation about poison ivy. To begin with, the name itself is misleading. The plant is neither a poison nor an ivy. *Rhus toxicodendron* is a member of the sumac family. Approximately seven out of ten people are allergic to it, but the plant is otherwise harmless. The weepy, itching skin eruption called "poison ivy" is a type of allergic contact dermatitis.

This chapter deals specifically with poison ivy, but the principles apply to all types of contact dermatitis, whether due to plants, makeup, shoes, or jewelry (Chapter 28). The rashes and their treatment differ only in degree and location.

Although not everyone is affected by exposure to poison ivy, it is still remarkable that the percentage is so high. By comparison, a cosmetic that caused one allergic reaction in every 1,000 users would be quickly removed from the market. Poison ivy allergy usually develops in childhood but may appear at any time in life. Attacks of poison ivy tend to be less severe and less frequent as one grows older, probably because one has less contact with the plant.

Poison ivy is a hardy plant found worldwide. In America, only the West Coast is free of it. (This area has a related species, poison oak.) The plant's well-known triads of shiny leaves are coated with an oil. You get poison ivy only when and where this oil touches and penetrates your skin. Usually this happens when you brush against the plant. If you handle poison ivy, you may not get a rash on your palms, where the thick skin is an excellent barrier, but only on other body areas you subsequently touch before washing the oil off your hands. The face is especially susceptible. It is also possible to get poison ivy by touching something else that has recently been in contact with the plant, such as clothing or a dog's fur. And it is possible to get a severe case by standing near a fire in which the plant is burning, because the oil reaches all the exposed skin in the smoke particles. Clearly, it may be difficult to discover exactly how you were exposed to poison ivy.

Once the oil is on your skin, it must remain there long enough to penetrate through the dead outer layer. Thorough washing within ten or twenty minutes of touching the plant may prevent the rash. It is always worthwhile to wash at least your hands after possible exposure to poison ivy, even if more than twenty minutes have elapsed, in order to remove oil that you might inadvertently spread to other areas.

After the oil has entered the skin, it usually takes two or three days for the rash to appear. Tuesday is a big day for poison ivy in a dermatologist's office, because so many people go hiking or picnicking on the weekend.

The oil has washed or worn off the skin long before the rash appears. Once present, the rash cannot spread either to other people or to other areas on your own

165

body. This is very difficult for people to accept, because they know that at first only a small area is involved, but after a day or two of scratching usually much more skin has blistered. This does *not* mean the blister fluid is contagious, as it is in certain viral and bacterial infections. The fluid is the same as that in blisters that develop after a burn and is simply the body's response to a local injury. The confusion arises because the skin that had the greatest exposure to the oil or that has the thinnest barrier layer develops the rash first. Areas that absorbed less oil are involved later and less severely. Scratching poison ivy is not helpful, but it does *not* spread the rash.

In general, a severe case of poison ivy begins sooner after exposure than a mild case — perhaps in one day instead of two or three. In a day or less, it evolves from a faint red itchy patch to large blisters. A mild case may never blister. Untreated, a severe case may last three weeks or more, although improvement always begins within the first week. A very mild case may disappear in a few days.

What can be done about poison ivy? As always, prevention is better than any treatment. Learn to recognize the plant and avoid it. When you are in places likely to harbor poison ivy, wear protective clothing and wash as soon as possible afterward.

If poison ivy develops despite your precautions, try to assess its severity early in the course. Swollen eyes on the first day, for example, are a bad omen. If the eruption is extensive and rapidly progressive or if you have a recent history of severe poison ivy, see your doctor.

Steroid pills or shots can completely block the allergic reaction and restore the skin to its normal state in a day or so, but the longer the rash has been present, the less effective they can be. Steroid medication is very potent and prolonged use carries several potential side effects, such as aggravation of diabetes, high blood pressure, or ulcers. It is used only in very severe cases of poison ivy and only if the prescribing physician feels there are no undue risks for the patient involved. Still, most dermatologists feel that the small risk of this therapy is justified in otherwise healthy people who would be forced to lose time from school or work by the full-blown eruption. If steroids are prescribed, they must be continued until the allergic reaction has subsided, usually in about two weeks. If the medicine is stopped prematurely, the rash quickly reappears.

If poison ivy is not severe enough to warrant steroid pills or shots, it may still be alleviated somewhat by frequent application of a steroid cream during the first few days. Such creams should not be used unless your doctor has prescribed them specifically for *this* eruption, because steroids worsen some conditions that you may have mistaken for poison ivy.

The two major problems with fully developed poison ivy are itching and weeping of the blisters. Chapter 20 suggests several ways to relieve itching. A lotion such as calamine is especially helpful, since it is both drying and soothing. Products that contain a topical anesthetic should be avoided, since they may produce their own allergic reaction. Chapter 39 describes how to hasten drying of blisters. In addition to those measures, a soft dry cloth, absorbent cotton, or gauze pads should be placed between opposing involved skin surfaces, such as in finger and toe webs or under the arm. Replace the material as often as necessary to keep the area comfortable.

Some physicians have attempted to "desensitize"

people with severe poison ivy allergy by feeding them plant extracts frequently in small amounts. The theoretic basis of this approach is sound, but it results in a very itchy bottom more often than in immunity to poison ivy.

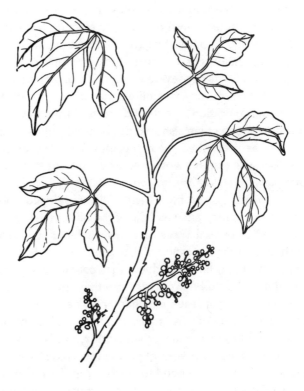

Don't tread on me!

28
Contact Dermatitis

This term refers either to irritant or to allergic reactions. In both cases, something that touches the skin causes a red, itchy, sometimes blistering rash to appear in the area of contact after a delay of several hours to several days. Untreated, the rash may last for days or weeks.

Irritant contact dermatitis is caused by substances such as strong acids or harsh chemicals; anyone who touches the substance long enough or often enough develops a rash. The origin of such rashes is rarely a mystery to the people who get them.

Allergic contact dermatitis may be caused by anything but appears only in people who are allergic to that substance. It is often difficult to determine exactly what has caused the rash. For example, if ingredient X is present in a certain lipstick or in a certain food coloring, a woman allergic to X might then develop a rash frequently on the lips or occasionally on the hands after baking. The "common denominator" may be hard to identify.

Some substances are very potent allergens. Poison ivy (Chapter 27), for instance, causes allergic reactions in a majority of people who are exposed. Most common allergens affect only one person in several thousand.

Contact dermatitis is suspect if a rash has an unusual pattern. A rash across the forehead may be due to a hatband or hair spray; a red itchy patch on the thigh may be due to keys carried in a trouser pocket. The only clue to the cause of allergic contact dermatitis is its location and pattern. Except for severity, the rashes are identical, whether produced by poison ivy or by toothpaste.

Anyone can develop an allergy. Once you are allergic to something, the sensitivity usually persists for life.

The only true solution to the problem of recurring contact dermatitis is to identify the exact substance responsible and then to avoid it. Some people succeed in this detective work, but often the culprit is still unknown after months of keeping lists and changing brands. At that point it is wise to consult a dermatologist, who can sometimes identify the allergy from the location of the rash and from information about work or hobbies and can also perform patch tests. In this procedure, suspected chemicals and common allergens are placed on a small area of skin for two or three days so that a rash can develop from any to which an allergy exists. The doctor examines the skin at the end of the test period and correlates the results with the rashes previously experienced. If the causative substance is identified, the doctor can provide a list of products that must be avoided and, finally, can treat the contact dermatitis itself.

This discussion implies that contact dermatitis is a chronic, low-grade problem. Usually it is, but the eruption may be quite devastating and explosive in onset. Chapter 27 discusses how to judge the severity of a developing reaction, when to consult a physician, and the medications available for contact dermatitis.

HAND ECZEMA

Hand eczema is not a specific disease but simply eczema affecting the hands. It has many other names, most referring to the occupation of the affected person rather than to the actual cause of the eczema: housewives' eczema, surgeons' hands, dishpan hands. It is the most frequent dermatitis among industrial workers. Its causes are many, because hands get into everything. Many cases are at least in part a form of contact dermatitis (see Chapter 28). Common underlying factors are environmental — low humidity, repeated exposure to mildly irritating chemicals, frequent hand-washing, and a tendency to develop allergies.

One type of hand eczema is rarely attributable to specific allergies. It is sometimes called *dyshidrotic eczema*, a misnomer based on the incorrect theory that lesions were due to faulty sweat secretion. Its cause is unknown, but attacks are more common and often more severe at times of emotional stress. Tiny blisters appear along the edges of the palms, fingers, and occasionally the soles. At first, the involved skin surface resembles tapioca, but later it becomes red, weepy, or scaly. Itching may be mild or severe or, in advanced cases, masked by pain due to deep cracks in the skin folds or superimposed bacterial infection.

Principles of treatment are the same for hand eczema as for generalized eczema. When exacerbating

171

factors can be avoided, response to therapy is often dramatic. Emotional stress appears to make hand eczema more difficult to tolerate or treat. Chronic hand eczema requires the attention of a dermatologist.

29

Seborrhea and Seborrheic Dermatitis

Seborrhea means excess oil or sebum production by the oil glands associated with hair follicles. This causes a greasy complexion. The term "seborrheic dermatitis" implies inflammation in skin caused by this excess oil production. In fact, the cause of seborrheic dermatitis is unknown. Most people with this disorder have only faint redness and scaling of the facial creases and hair-bearing areas such as the scalp, eyebrows, and, in men, the chest. The condition may cause mild itching. A predisposition toward seborrheic dermatitis is inborn. Affected infants have cradle cap, a form of dandruff, and a tendency to develop severe diaper rashes. After infancy, dandruff may persist through childhood but usually disappears until adolescence. Involvement of areas other than the scalp may then occur gradually during adulthood. Seborrheic dermatitis is rarely a significant problem.

Neither seborrhea nor seborrheic dermatitis can be "cured," but usually each is easily controlled. Washing the face with a drying soap two or three times daily prevents oil from accumulating on the skin surface (see Chapter 23). Wiping with a damp face cloth in mid-

morning and midafternoon is less drying and also removes the "shine" caused by excess skin oil. Redness
and scaling on the face disappear with daily use of a
steroid cream. This medicine *must* be prescribed by
your physician. A steroid cream should *never be used,
especially on the face or for long periods of time, unless it is
prescribed for that purpose.* The more common, more expensive, and more potent creams may produce permanent thinning of the skin and prominence of the blood
vessels after only a few months of regular use. Safe and
less expensive steroids such as hydrocortisone are
available for seborrheic dermatitis. The treatment of
dandruff associated with seborrheic dermatitis is discussed in Chapter 15.

Seborrhea and Seborrheic Dermatitis

30
Bacterial
Infections

IMPETIGO

Impetigo is a type of superficial skin infection caused by streptococci and/or staphylococci. Lesions have a characteristic golden-yellow crust, are usually small, and may occur in clusters. They are not painful and do not cause fever or malaise.

Impetigo frequently begins in damaged skin. Any open, weeping area of skin is quickly invaded by bacteria. If a sufficient number of streptococci are present, the lesion becomes redder, slightly tender or itchy, develops a yellow crust, and is said to be *impetiginized*. Frequently insect bites, scratches, burns, or abrasions lead to this superficial infection. Even when impetigo appears to begin on normal skin, there may have been preceding minor trauma. Small epidemics of impetigo may occur, especially in groups of children at, say, a camp or day-care center, or in several members of a family.

Rheumatic fever, which sometimes follows streptococcal throat infections, is fortunately not a complication of impetigo, but a form of kidney damage called *acute glomerulonephritis* does occur occasionally. Glomerulonephritis is an indirect result of the body's reaction to invading bacteria but may be far more serious than the infection itself. In some parts of the southern United States, more than half of all cases are preceded by impetigo.

Impetigo usually heals without treatment after a few weeks and never leaves a scar. Since the infection is very superficial and usually involves only a small area, it is tempting just to ignore it. However, antibiotic treatment causes the lesions to heal more rapidly, reduces spread to other people and the risk of recurrence, and probably lessens the risk of acute glomerulonephritis.

Very small areas can be treated with a topical antibiotic ointment such as bacitracin, available without prescription. Gently remove the crusts with soap and water two or three times daily and immediately apply a small amount of ointment. If the lesion is larger than a fifty-cent piece, it usually requires a systemic rather than topical antibiotic. Your doctor can prescribe penicillin, erythromycin, or an acceptable alternate drug. Family members and medical attendants should wash thoroughly with an antibacterial soap after treating a person with impetigo. A person with impetigo should not share towels, bed linen, or other intimate articles until the lesions have healed. If impetigo occurs repeatedly in a family or other small group, everyone should be examined by a doctor, since people who harbor the bacteria in their noses, throats, or other areas without becoming ill may still spread infection to others.

Infection around hair follicles is called *folliculitis*. It can occur anywhere on the body but most commonly occurs on the buttocks and thighs. Often many hairs are involved simultaneously or sequentially. The small pustules or pimples, each at the base of a hair, usually heal uneventfully in a week or less. In rare cases, folliculitis is more severe, lasts longer, and causes permanent loss of the involved hairs.

Prolonged wetness of the skin, chronic rubbing or chafing, poor aeration, and frequent contact with heavy oils or grease are sometimes factors in folliculitis. Obesity, diabetes, and poor resistance to infection also increase the risk, but most people with folliculitis are otherwise completely healthy.

Daily use of an antibacterial soap (such as Dial® or Zest®), pHisoHex®, or Betadine® in lieu of a standard bath soap may decrease future lesions by temporarily diminishing the population of bacteria on the skin surface. Such washing should continue for at least a month. If bothersome lesions persist, a physician can check for underlying problems and prescribe a two-week course of an appropriate antibiotic. However, despite the best therapy, low-grade folliculitis sometimes persists.

BOILS: FURUNCLES AND CARBUNCLES

A *furuncle* is an acute, often painful abscess located around a hair follicle. The infection is usually due to staphylococci. A sty, which surrounds an eyelash, is a common example, but boils may occur anywhere. A *carbuncle* is a group of interconnecting furuncles. These lesions may be considered a severe form of folliculitis and have the same predisposing factors.

Boils begin as firm, tender, red swellings that rapidly enlarge. After several days they become boggy and "point," forming a white or yellow pustule near the skin surface. Usually the lesions rupture spontaneously and discharge thick pus tinged with blood. Rupture relieves the pain and allows healing to begin. Carbuncles may cause scarring, but simple boils usually disappear without a trace in a week or two.

Small boils do not need any treatment. Large or extensive lesions, which produce fever, pain, swollen lymph glands, and general malaise, often require a visit to a local emergency room or physician's office.

For home treatment, apply warm compresses to relieve the pain and hasten "pointing." Soak a soft cloth in warm water, then hold it against the lesion until the cloth cools. Apply such compresses continuously for fifteen or twenty minutes at least four times daily. The cloth should not be used by other people until it has been washed in boiling water for five minutes or in the hot cycle of a washing machine. Once a boil has matured, the central pustule can be nicked with a freshly opened razor blade or other sterile instrument, so the lesion can drain. Do *not* attempt to do this unless you are comfortable with the procedure and have the proper equipment. Do *not* use a pin, razor, or knife blade heated in a match flame. Often the cutting surface is not sterile, and, moreover, carbon particles from the flame may be introduced into the skin, leaving a permanent black tattoo. Do not attempt to drain a boil before it points, since this may aggravate the infection. Consult your doctor about a boil on the first day if the infection promises to be severe, so that an appropriate antibiotic can be prescribed to lessen inflammation and discomfort. If the lesion is already fully developed, an antibiotic is nearly useless. Your doctor can also drain a boil that has pointed and is better equipped to do this than you are. Especially if boils are large or located in awkward areas, get professional help. Because diabetes and other diseases are sometimes associated with boils, your doctor may also wish to order blood and urine tests.

People with frequent boils should be checked at least once for the possibility of an underlying illness, but usually no reason for the infections is found. Rigorous personal hygiene is the best defense against future lesions because this reduces and alters the bacteria on the skin. Use antibacterial soaps or cleansers, described in the preceding section. Bacitracin ointment can be applied just inside the nostrils daily. This destroys a reservoir of bacteria that is not exposed to soap. Wash all fingernails with a brush daily. Shave with a disposable razor and, preferably, discard it after each shave. When lesions are active, do not share towels, washcloths, or other personal articles.

31
Cold Sores

Cold sores, also called fever blisters, are an infection caused by *herpes virus hominis*. The medical term for these infections is *herpes simplex*.

The virus can be found almost everywhere in our environment, and more than half the population has been infected at some time. The virus infects only human beings.

Infection begins when the herpes virus enters through a small break in the skin. The body's first encounter with the virus may go unnoticed or may produce extensive painful blistering. These infections often occur inside the mouth or on the genitalia, since it is easiest for the virus to penetrate the skin barrier in these areas. Primary infections in the mouth are most common in small children; the pain may interfere with eating for several days. Genital infection occurs most often in young adults. Genital herpes simplex, usually acquired through sexual contact, is discussed in Chapters 32 and 36.

After the primary infection, which heals without treatment in about two weeks, the virus appears to withdraw from the site of original infection to a nearby nerve and to remain there indefinitely. The body's immune defenses hold the virus at bay inside the nerve until times of stress, such as a severe illness or even a mild cold, when the virus apparently overwhelms the body's preoccupied immune defenses and reappears. The reactivated virus travels along a branch of the infected nerve to a specific skin site. Each episode occurs in the same general area, usually on the lip, near the site of primary infection. Herpes simplex may occur anywhere, however.

These recurrent infections are usually mild. The involved area often feels numb or tender for several hours. Then a small cluster of blisters appears. There may be swelling in the skin and nearby lymph nodes. The blisters soon break, crusts form, and the lesion gradually heals after one to two weeks. Herpes simplex never scars.

It is impossible to predict how many times or how frequently a cold sore will appear. Some people have only one attack in a lifetime; others have active infections every few weeks for years. A few unfortunate women get herpes simplex with each menstrual period. In other people, a sunburn or fever or even nervous tension precipitates an attack.

In the quiescent period between attacks, the virus causes no problem for the infected person and is not contagious to others. The blisters of active herpes simplex are highly contagious to others, however. Lesions remain contagious until the blisters are completely dry, usually for two or three days in recurrent attacks.

There are two potential complications of herpes simplex. One is *herpes keratitis,* a painful infection involving the cornea of the eye, that can lead to blindness. The eye becomes inflamed and feels as if a particle of dirt were trapped under the lid. *If such eye*

181

symptoms begin when a cold sore is present, see an ophthalmologist immediately. He or she can perform a special examination to identify the infection and can prescribe medication to cure it before permanent damage occurs. *Secondly, never use a steroid medication in or near the eyes during a herpes attack.* Steroids decrease inflammation and are occasionally even prescribed to treat cold sores, but they also make it much easier for the virus to infect the eye. Finally, if recurrent herpes simplex lesions occur near the eyes, consult an ophthalmologist before eye symptoms appear. He may advise an antiviral medication for the eyes during each attack to lower the risk of keratitis.

The second complication affects only people with eczema or a history of eczema. In these people, the herpes virus can spread from a cold sore and cause blistering lesions over much of the body surface, even if the skin is free of eczema at the time. Spread need not occur with each attack of herpes but can be devastating when it does. If possible, people with eczema should avoid being exposed to herpes infection in the first place. If spread begins, they should seek medical attention immediately so that a superimposed bacterial infection can be prevented. Steroid creams or ointments being used for the eczema itself should be discontinued while a cold sore is present, since these medications may facilitate the spread of virus.

In infants and in people with severe illnesses, herpes infections can involve the lungs, brain, and other internal organs, as well as the skin. Such infections are often fatal. People with poor resistance to infection must be carefully protected from herpes virus; there is no effective treatment once infection begins.

Despite these dire possibilities, herpes simplex, in a basically healthy person, is very rarely more than a nuisance. Even a harmless infection can be annoying, however, especially if it occurs frequently. It may be a major inconvenience, as well as being unsightly. Because herpes simplex is so common and so unpopular, numerous therapies have been devised. Each new treatment is greeted enthusiastically by both patients and doctors; each has a group of devotees who swear it works for them. Unfortunately, so far no treatment has been scientifically proved to speed healing or to reduce the frequency of cold sores. On the other hand, a person bothered by cold sores has little to lose by trying to treat the infection.

There are several products on the market such as Stoxil® and Herplex® that contain *idoxuridine,* an antiviral drug effective against herpes infections of the eye. Recommended usage is three times daily until healing occurs. However, the drug penetrates into the skin so poorly that it cannot reach the living virus and is therefore ineffective for skin lesions.

Some doctors recommend a steroid cream such as Lidex® or Halog® for the brief period before blisters appear, when the skin begins to burn or tingle. They believe that hourly applications to that site can sometimes abort developing infection. Use of the cream should be stopped if blisters appear.

Rubbing alcohol, an acne lotion, or salt-water compresses (see Chapter 39) may be applied four to six times daily to the blisters to hasten drying. Dabbing the anesthetic ether on herpes simplex lesions has the same rationale but is impractical, since liquid ether is highly flammable and explosive.

Antibacterial ointments such as bacitracin, applied two or three times daily, help by preventing bacterial infection of the lesion but do not kill the virus.

If sunburn provokes the cold sores, regular use of a

sunscreen such as PreSun® or Pabanol® on the face may prevent lesions and is advisable on other grounds in any case (see Chapter 12).

Dye and light treatments, vaccinations, and a variety of other therapies for herpes simplex are still controversial, experimental, and not worth the expense of long trips or frequent professional consultations. In the long run, many people are less bothered by their cold sores than by the colds that may have provoked them. Rightly so.

Cold Sores

32

Genital Herpes Simplex
(Herpes Progenitalis)

Infection with herpes virus hominis may occur any-where on the body. Lesions on the genitalia are in-creasingly common, and herpes probably is the number two venereal disease in America today. The infection, which is identical to cold sores except in lo-cation and mode of spread, is fully discussed in Chap-ter 31. This chapter focuses on the problems peculiar to genital herpes simplex.

The first or primary infection with herpes simplex occurs about thirty hours after exposure and may be excruciatingly painful. The entire head of the penis in men and the much larger area between the legs in women may develop small blisters. The blisters quickly break, leaving a weepy, painful surface that usually requires at least three weeks to heal. Lymph nodes in the groin become swollen and tender. Fever is common. Especially in women, where the raw surfaces rub against each other, walking or even sitting may be impossible. Pain and swelling may prevent urination. These symptoms bring most people to a doctor's office or hospital emergency ward within a day or two.

There is no cure for herpes simplex itself. However,

prescription medications for pain relief and for prevention or treatment of a superimposed bacterial infection are most helpful. Frequent sitz baths at home also lessen the discomfort. Fill the tub with enough warm water to submerge the infected area and soak for twenty minutes three to six times daily. It is less painful to pass urine while sitting in the tub, because the bath water dilutes and carries away the usually acid wastes. After urinating, drain and refill the tub to cleanse the skin. After each sitz bath, spray Americaine® or another local anesthetic on the raw areas. The numbing effect lasts one or two hours and may allow some normal activities. These sprays should be used only for very severe pain, however, since allergies may develop and then cause new problems (see Chapter 20). During the time the anesthetic is working, care must be taken not to traumatize the insensitive area by scratching, pressing, or rubbing. When anesthesia is no longer required, petrolatum or other bland ointment may be applied gently to protect the area from irritation by clothing or opposing skin surfaces. Exposing the infected area to the air hastens drying and hence healing. Since severe herpes simplex often restricts a person to bed, this is not as difficult as it sounds. Uncircumsized men can retract their foreskins; women can lie on their backs with knees apart. Fifteen minutes four times daily is sufficient, but longer exposure is better.

Recurrent herpes simplex is usually mild, an annoyance that lasts from two to ten days. There is no effective method of decreasing the number or frequency of attacks. The public health problem here is that lack of pain allows a person to remain sexually active. Because herpes simplex is highly contagious when lesions are present, the infection spreads rapidly from person to

Genital Herpes Simplex (Herpes Progenitalis)

person. Abstinence for the period that lesions are visible is the only way to prevent spread of the virus. The first four days are the most critical.

Genital herpes simplex has a special significance in pregnant women, since infants exposed to the virus at birth may develop overwhelming infection. For this reason, obstetricians and infectious disease experts prefer a cesarean section to vaginal delivery if lesions are present when labor begins. An expectant mother with recurrent herpes simplex should notify her physician of the infection. Fortunately, herpes simplex is rare in the final weeks of pregnancy.

Herpes simplex has recently received a great deal of publicity because of a possible link with cervical cancer. People of both sexes are understandably frightened by such reports. It is important to emphasize that herpes simplex has never been shown to cause cancer in anyone. Cancer of the cervix is more common among women who have had genital herpes, but the statistical association of these problems does not establish a cause and effect relationship. Routine annual gynecologic examinations, recommended for all women over age thirty in any case, are ample precaution for women with recurrent herpes simplex. Routine checkups every five years are adequate for affected men.

Genital Herpes Simplex (Herpes Progenitalis)

33
Yeast
Infections

The yeast *Candida albicans* is a normal inhabitant of the mouth, the large intestine, and the vagina. When the body's ecologic balance is disturbed, it may overgrow or spread to the skin surface and cause infection. *Candidiasis* and *moniliasis* are medical terms for these infections.

Yeast infection may be suspected from its appearance, but diagnosis usually requires microscopic examination of skin scrapings. This chapter complements, but does not replace, a visit to a physician who can do the necessary tests and then prescribe appropriate medication.

Yeasts love warmth, moisture, and glucose (sugar). These factors largely determine which people develop moniliasis and where the infections occur. The perfect candidate is an obese pregnant diabetic woman, living in a warm climate and being treated with antibiotics for a bacterial infection. Most people with moniliasis have one or more of these risk factors. Yeasts multiply quickly in deep sweaty skin folds, especially if the levels of sugar in the body fluids are high. This causes *monilial intertrigo:* large shiny red itchy areas with a sharp border, sometimes surrounded by small red spots or pimples, most often in the groin or under the breasts. Antibiotics, taken for whatever reason, kill many of the bacteria that normally live on the skin surface and hence remove the yeast's competitors for food and space. Pregnancy (or birth control pills) increases the amount of sugar in vaginal tissues and so further facilitates local yeast overgrowth, causing an itchy, creamy vaginal discharge.

Yeast infections also occur in normal infants, in part because the body's immune defenses are poorly developed at this age. These infections are usually in the diaper area, which is warm and moist most of the time and repeatedly covered with yeast-containing fecal material. *Thrush* (significant moniliasis of the mouth or oral cavity) is uncommon unless the baby has received antibiotics. A seeming anomaly among settings for yeast infections is the fold at the base of the fingernail. This area may remain slightly red, swollen, and tender for years as a result of low-grade moniliasis in people such as dishwashers and bartenders whose hands are frequently in water (see Chapter 18).

Many cases of moniliasis can be cured simply by depriving the yeast of warmth and moisture. A treatment regimen that does not do this usually fails. Medications containing *nystatin* (Mycostatin®, Mycolog®) or any of several recently developed drugs are very helpful but are not a substitute for correcting the factors underlying a yeast infection. Air conditioning, loose clothing, and weight loss often make the difference between cure of monilial intertrigo and immediate relapse. Direct exposure of infected areas to a fan for ten minutes several times daily is ideal therapy. An absorbent powder such as Zeasorb® or baby powder may then be sprinkled on the skin. Cornstarch is not an ap-

189

propriate substitute since it is nourishment for yeast. In cases of genital moniliasis, regular sex partners should also be treated to prevent "Ping-Pong" — back and forth — infections. The most effective medicines will not cure a nailfold infection unless the hands are kept dry. Protective rubber gloves with cotton liners must be worn when working with water or moist substances.

A person with frequent or persistent yeast infections should have a blood or urine test to check for diabetes, since susceptibility to yeast may be an early and correctable sign of this condition.

Yeast Infections

34
Lice
(Pediculosis)

Lice are blood-sucking wingless insects that live on or near the skin. There they eat, multiply, and deposit excrement. Lice pass from person to person during close contact. In crowded, unsanitary conditions, pediculosis is rampant; it never completely disappears from society. Three kinds of lice parasitize man. They differ in appearance and in preferred location on the skin.

Head and body lice are quite similar. The female is about 1/6 inch long and the male is slightly smaller. Each female lays about eight eggs daily. The eggs hatch in a week or so and require another eight days to mature.

The head louse usually remains on the scalp or beard area. The infestation causes severe itching. Scratching may be so intense that scratch marks, secondary bacterial infection, and swollen lymph glands mask the condition. It is unusual to see lice on the scalp, but egg sacks, called "nits," can be seen rather easily. They are tiny, white knots that resemble dandruff flakes but are firmly attached to the hair shaft near the scalp. The infestation spreads to others via combs, brushes, towels, or hats. It is quite contagious and remains a common problem among school children even in the "best" neighborhoods.

The body louse lives in the seams of clothing and lays its eggs there. It visits the skin only for a blood meal, then returns to the clothing. The only evidence of its presence is bites, often grouped in threes: "breakfast, lunch, and dinner." A louse prefers to feed at frequent intervals but can survive up to ten days between meals. Newborns can survive slightly longer. In any case, garments that have been stored for one month are not infested. The lice can be transferred from one person to another by direct contact or by way of clothing, bedding, or towels. Occasionally, outer garments also harbor living insects.

The pubic louse differs in appearance and habits from its cousins. It is rounder and has large clawlike pincers that make it resemble a tiny crab. Hence, the popular name for this infestation: "crabs." It prefers the region covered by pubic hair, although occasionally it infests eyelashes and underarm areas. These crab lice cling constantly to the skin, feeding intermittently, and laying eggs that appear as nits. This type of lice is most often spread by sexual contact, but can also be contracted from bed linen, towels, or, rarely, toilet seats. Pubic lice are far more common than head or body lice in America today.

How can you know if you have lice? People infested with lice itch. Often their friends, families, and sexual partners also itch. However, itchiness is much more common than pediculosis. Just thinking about lice makes many people itch. But everyone who is itching because of lice has something visible on the skin — lice, nits, bites, or specks of excrement. You can see these signs, and your doctor can easily confirm the

192

diagnosis. The signs are always there; they do not come and go without treatment.

If you believe you have lice, see your doctor. Most effective treatments require a physician's prescription, and often separate medication is needed for relief of the itching or for secondary infection. And there is always the possibility that you may be wrong. Many people mistake a speck of dirt or lint for lice. If you treat yourself before being examined by your physician, it may be very difficult to unravel the problem later, if self-treatment fails.

Treatment for pediculosis is easy. Any of several creams, shampoos, or lotions may be applied to the affected areas according to instructions, usually only once. These medications kill all the insects immediately, but the egg sacks enclosing unborn lice may remain attached to the hairs, despite adequate treatment. These dead nits are harmless and can be ignored, but are easily removed with a special comb designed for this use and available in most drug stores. In order to loosen the nits, wet the hair with vinegar, cover with a towel for an hour, comb thoroughly, and shampoo. With modern treatment, shaving the head or other hair-bearing areas is unnecessary. Because the chemicals in the various lotions and shampoos are irritants and poisons, they must not be used excessively, especially in children. If you are not cured by the recommended dose, do not repeat it without consulting your doctor again.

Itching is not caused by the insects themselves, but rather by the body's allergic response to them. Hence, itching may persist for many days after all the lice are gone. After completing the therapy, wash all clothing, bedding, towels, and the like that might contain insects or nits and that you plan to use within the maximum possible period of contagion. This period is one month for body lice and about two weeks for head lice and pubic lice. Sometimes it is impossible to wash or to avoid all possibly contaminated articles. Do the best you can. Intimate friends of a person with pediculosis should be observed carefully for several weeks and treated immediately if infestation appears. For this reason, school authorities must be informed if a child is infested.

Lice (Pediculosis)

35
Scabies

The mite *Sarcoptes scabiei* is responsible for "the seven-year itch" that has plagued countless thousands, purportedly including Napoleon, throughout history. The female is barely visible to the naked eye but appears menacing under the microscope. She spends her days burrowing just below the skin surface. There she eats, defecates, mates with the smaller males, and lays three or four eggs per day. The eggs hatch and begin a new cycle in less than a week. At first, the infestation causes no symptoms, but eventually the unfortunate host becomes allergic to the insects. After this happens, a person experiences severe itching whenever the mite enters the skin. Eventually itching is continuous and may affect most of the body. Nodules, blisters, or minute burrows appear on the skin and these lesions are often scratched. The mites seem particularly fond of the webspaces between fingers, the wrists, and thighs and buttocks, and the head of the penis. The face and scalp are not involved except in some small children.

Scabies is almost always acquired through intimate contact with infested people. In adults, it is often a venereal disease. Rarely are contaminated clothing, bedding, furniture, or towels responsible. Off the skin, the mites cannot survive for more than two days.

Even if you have good reason to suspect scabies, it is foolish to treat yourself without consulting a physician. Definite diagnosis is difficult, even for experts. Misdiagnosis is easy, and improper self-treatment can create weeks or months of itchy uncertainty.

The approach to diagnosis and therapy, the effective medications, and the problems of incorrect treatment are very similar for infestation with either mites and lice (see Chapter 34). The major differences are that scabies usually require slightly more therapy than pediculosis, two or three applications of cream instead of one; that the "period of contagion" is shorter, only two days rather than two to four weeks; and that it is usually advisable to treat all intimate contacts of an infested person immediately, rather than when symptoms appear.

36
Venereal Diseases

Anyone can get venereal disease. Many people do: rich and poor, college professors and illiterates, infants and grandparents, as well as young adults.

The subject of VD may seem out of place in a book about skin disorders. Many people are not aware that dermatologists as well as infectious disease specialists and gynecologists are centrally involved in the diagnosis and treatment of these conditions. In fact, most VD treatment programs today are headed by a dermatologist, and until 1955 physicians trained in skin diseases were certified by the Board of Dermatology and Syphilology. Only recently have laboratory tests in part replaced examination of the skin in the diagnosis of syphilis, gonorrhea, and other disorders.

Man's attitude toward VD is a complicated mixture of his attitude toward sex and his emotional reactions to diseases that affect the skin. The usual fear of contagion and the feeling of shame that accompany a skin lesion are magnified when the skin disease is a result of sexual communication or when its presence limits further sexual activity. Those who consider sex sinful and vulgar see VD as the ugliest end of an untouchable

197

spectrum; those who see sex as romantic and beautiful view VD as a spoiler and interrupter. The primitive view of disease as retribution is magnified when the disease involves the genitalia. Victims of VD are beneath contempt. Because of other societal prejudices, this judgmental attitude is magnified if the victim is a female, a black, or a homosexual. Such attitudes prevent open dissemination of medical information and make persons with VD reluctant to seek medical attention. This is tragic because VD is treatable, its spread is preventable, and its effects are avoidable.

The word "venereal" is derived from Venus, the Roman goddess of love. There are five classic venereal diseases, some now quite rare, but the term may be used for any contagious disease transmitted during sexual intercourse. Common examples at this time include herpes simplex, moniliasis (yeast infections), condyloma accuminata (venereal warts), pediculosis (lice), and scabies (see Chapters 32–37). The mode of spread is the only common bond among the venereal diseases.

This chapter discusses the more common types of VD and the appearance of these diseases on the skin. There are many misconceptions about VD in our society, despite extensive public health education efforts. First, to get VD, you must have skin-to-skin contact with a lesion of an infected person. You do not get VD from toilet seats or by shaking hands. There are extremely few exceptions to this rule. Second, not all skin lesions on the genitalia are venereal disease. Many common noncontagious disorders occur in this area. Conversely, venereal lesions may occur almost anywhere, although the genitalia are affected most often. Third, a physician will not always correctly diagnose VD unless you mention the possibility. Doc-

198

tors, like everyone else, assume unconsciously that "nice people" cannot get such infections. If you are worried about VD, do not try to convince your physician that your symptoms are due to a virus or an allergy. Tell the truth, so that the doctor may perform the proper tests or, if you are mistakenly concerned, provide reassurance.

Paradoxically, these "dirty" diseases are caused by very fastidious germs. The microorganisms of VD quickly die if removed from warm moist areas such as the mouth, vagina, anus, or head of the penis. This prerequisite assures that the diseases are transferred only through intimate contact. Conventions of dress and behavioral taboos in civilized Western society leave sexual intercourse as the only form of body contact adequate for the spread of these organisms.

We have already stressed that VD is acquired by intimate contact with a lesion of an infected person. Often, however, the lesion is inconspicuous. A sore located under the penile foreskin, within the vagina, in the anal canal, or in the back of the throat may not be noticed even by an observant sexual partner, or indeed by the infected person. Similarly, a slight discharge from the penis or vagina may be accepted as normal.

With the exception of condoms, birth control devices do nothing to prevent the spread of VD. Condoms offer some protection, but the diseases are still frequently transmitted either to or from male users.

How can you know if you have a venereal disease? If you are sexually active, you may be infected, even if you have no symptoms. In general, the larger the number of sexual partners, the greater the risk of exposure. But no sexually active person is safe from VD. Women especially may become infected with syphilis, gonorrhea, or venereal warts and never realize that anything

199

is wrong. Such infections are detected only through routine screening examinations or because sexual partners develop symptoms and seek medical assistance. Much more often, however, symptoms of VD develop within days or a few weeks after the initial infection. The symptoms of the common venereal diseases are discussed in their respective subsections.

A properly equipped physician can virtually always detect VD, but only by performing the correct tests. VD clinics are ideally equipped for the detection and treatment of these diseases but are not always available, and embarrassment or distaste unfortunately discourages many people from using these facilities. If you seek help in another setting, be sure the physician understands your concern about VD. Microscopic examinations may be performed on certain skin lesions and discharges within minutes to determine whether VD exists. In other cases, biopsies, bacterial cultures, or blood tests must be done, and diagnosis must be deferred for several days. Only in rare situations is VD difficult to diagnose, however.

Treatment depends on the type of VD, the stage of the disease, and on the possibility that allergies or other problems preclude the use of the standard antibiotics. Usually treatment consists of one or two antibiotic injections. Penicillin is the drug of choice for treating both syphilis and gonorrhea, but a different preparation and regimen must be used for each disease. Other antibiotics are available for people allergic to penicillin. After treatment, bacterial cultures or blood tests are repeated to be sure the infection is cured. All recent sexual partners must also be examined. This aspect of VD treatment is essential to controlling the spread of infection and is required by law.

200

Self-treatment almost never works. It is dangerous for the person who attempts it and is unfair to his or her contacts. No medication available without a doctor's prescription can cure VD. Even the correct medications fail unless used in exactly the right way. Since symptoms of VD normally come and go during the course of the disease, a person may believe the disease is cured when, in fact, it persists and will cause more trouble in the future.

Effective antibiotic treatment of VD is one of the miracles of modern medicine. Until the discovery of penicillin in the 1940s, the diagnosis of VD had the same impact as the diagnosis of cancer today. It virtually guaranteed suffering or deformity and not infrequently a shortened life span. Patients were treated with poisons that sometimes caused more illness than the VD itself.

SYPHILIS

Syphilis is a bacterial infection caused by the spirochete *Treponema pallidum*. Under the microscope, this organism looks like a long, thin corkscrew and moves with a graceful spiraling motion. Infection usually occurs during sexual contact but may be acquired by a fetus before birth from its infected mother or, very rarely, after birth by blood transfusion or other unusual circumstances. In some people, syphilis produces minor symptoms and then disappears forever without treatment; in others it causes serious illness and death. Syphilis is curable. If it is treated early, no permanent damage results.

Infection begins immediately after you touch a syphilitic lesion. Bacteria multiply locally in the skin, within hours enter the bloodstream and lymph channels, and soon are carried throughout the body. During this early invasion, there are no skin lesions or other evidence of infection. Blood tests are negative. This stage of the disease is called incubating syphilis and cannot be diagnosed.

The first lesion of syphilis occurs at the site of the original bacterial invasion, ten days to three months — usually about three weeks — after exposure. This lesion is the *syphilitic chancre*, and this stage of the disease is *primary* syphilis. The chancre is usually a painless, firm, slightly raised sore with a glistening surface. It is teeming with bacteria and is highly infectious. Usually a single sore appears on the genitalia, but chancres may occur anywhere, depending on where and how the original exposure occurred, and there may be more than one. Painless swelling of nearby lymph glands usually accompanies the chancre. If the chancre is on the genitalia, the enlarged glands are in the groin. Untreated, the chancre heals in one to three months. All evidence of infection disappears, even though syphilis is still present.

Primary syphilis can be diagnosed by examining moisture from the chancre surface with a special microscope. Blood tests for syphilis become positive a few days to a month after the chancre appears and so are frequently but not always diagnostic at this stage.

Weeks to months after the chancre heals, a widespread rash may appear. This is a *secondary* syphilis. In rare cases, the rash of secondary syphilis appears before the chancre heals. The lesions of secondary syphilis may be flat, raised, red or brown, easily visible or very subtle, itchy or symptomless, but in any one per-

202

son all the lesions are similar in appearance. They are scattered over the entire body surface and often involve the palms and soles. These lesions also contain bacteria but are much less contagious than the chancre of primary syphilis, except in moist areas like the mouth, vulva, or anus. Spotty, temporary hair loss on the scalp may accompany the rash; fever, weakness, and swollen lymph glands are common. Internal organs such as the liver, kidney, eye, or brain may be severely damaged in rare cases.

If untreated, the disease again disappears after weeks to months. You are still infected but look and feel well. The only evidence of syphilis is a positive blood test. This is *latent* syphilis. After two years, the disease is no longer contagious for others.

An experienced physician strongly suspects secondary syphilis when he sees the characteristic rash. Diagnosis is confirmed by the blood test for syphilis, which is always positive at this stage. A skin biopsy also reveals the diagnosis, but is rarely necessary.

Primary and secondary syphilis and the first year or so of latent syphilis make up the period of infectiousness. The disease may be transmitted during sexual intercourse or, if a woman becomes pregnant, to her unborn child. Appropriate therapy within this period is curative; all traces of the disease are eradicated and the blood test reverts to negative.

Without treatment, three outcomes are possible. In two-thirds of cases, syphilis seems to disappear. The person has no further symptoms of the disease. In half of these cases, even the blood test eventually returns to normal. In the remaining one-third of cases, *tertiary* syphilis appears. Slow, progressive destruction of tissue occurs, often after a lapse of many years. The disease may affect any organ. A person may become

203

demented, insane, deformed, or crippled. Death may result from involvement of the heart, brain, or other vital structure. Treatment at this stage may prevent further tissue destruction but cannot reverse existing damage. The blood test for syphilis usually remains positive.

Congenital syphilis is often an advanced disease, even though the infection has been present less than nine months. Some babies are stillborn. Others live to develop mental retardation, blindness, deafness, deformed bones and teeth, and many other tragic handicaps. Treatment after birth cannot prevent these problems, but adequate treatment of the infected mother during pregnancy may. For this reason, a blood test for syphilis is part of routine prenatal care.

GONORRHEA (GC, CLAP)

This infection is caused by bacteria called *Neisseria gonorrhoeae* or *gonococci*.

In men, infection usually begins two to five days after exposure, just inside the opening of the urethra on the tip of the penis. Urination may cause marked discomfort, and a penile discharge nearly always appears. The discharge may be clear but is more often cloudy white or yellow. The "drip" is usually most noticeable soon after awakening. While the discharge is present, GC is highly contagious to others. After several weeks, the drip disappears even without treatment, but the bacteria may then spread up the urethra or urine canal and into the prostate gland. Years later, scars may form that interfere with the passage of urine.

204

Gonorrhea can be recognized within minutes by microscopic examination of the urethral discharge. There is no blood test for GC. So if the discharge has already stopped, diagnosis is difficult.

Women with gonorrhea often have no symptoms during the early, contagious phase of the disease. Mild lower abdominal discomfort resembling menstrual cramps or a slight vaginal discharge may occur but can easily be overlooked. The initial infection usually involves the cervix. It may heal completely after several weeks or may spread upward, invading the uterus (womb), fallopian tubes, which lead to the ovaries, and even the lower abdomen. This type of infection is called *pelvic inflammatory disease* (PID). Acute PID causes high fever and severe pain. Most women must be hospitalized for relief of pain and for intravenous antibiotic therapy. Chronic or recurrent PID scars the pelvic organs and may cause sterility.

In women, gonorrhea usually must be diagnosed by bacterial cultures taken from the vagina and anus, where the organisms often spread even without anal intercourse. In advanced cases, routine cultures may be negative. Surgery may be necessary to find gonococci, buried in pelvic abscesses.

Like all VD, gonorrhea begins at the site of exposure. The penis and cervix are most common, but GC also occurs in the anus, in the throat, and very rarely elsewhere. Infants exposed to gonorrhea while passing through the birth canal frequently develop eye infections. Such infections caused blindness in many children before hospitals adopted the policy of putting antibacterial drops in the eyes of all newborns.

In both men and women untreated gonorrhea may also invade the bloodstream and spread throughout the body. In such cases, the person usually feels mildly

205

ill and has many painful joints and small red skin lesions with a central lake of pus scattered over the hands, forearms, and lower legs. This type of infection is potentially life-threatening.

In early cases, treatment of GC is easy and curative. In neglected cases, treatment may require hospitalization and often cannot correct the complications discussed above.

37
Venereal Warts
(Condyloma Accuminata)

Venereal warts are a viral infection of the skin on the genitalia that differ in appearance from standard warts (see Chapter 25). They form small bumps and later exuberant projections on the skin surface, usually on the tip of the penis or around the vaginal or anal opening. The two types of warts are probably caused by different viruses but might represent two different skin reactions to the same infection.

Like all warts, venereal warts are harmless but unsightly, sometimes uncomfortable, and, if untreated, tend to spread. They seem more contagious to others than warts on other parts of the body, perhaps because sexual intercourse provides greater exposure to the virus than do most types of human contact.

Warts are easily treated when small. They can be destroyed in a doctor's office by freezing with liquid nitrogen (see Chapter 25) or by painting with a harsh chemical, *podophyllin.* Treatments are moderately painful (but not as bad as you might imagine) and must be repeated every week or two until all warts are gone, in order to prevent relapse. One treatment is usually sufficient for scattered small warts, but months of therapy may be required for advanced cases.

Regular sexual partners should also be examined and treated to prevent "Ping-Pong" infections. Vaginal and rectal warts or small warts in any location are difficult to detect without special training and equipment, so such examinations are necessary even if no lesions are visible.

There are no long-term complications of venereal warts, and proper therapy does not produce scars.

Venereal Warts (Condyloma Accuminata)

38

Fungus
Infections

We are repulsed at the thought of a fungus infection,
yet well over half of us have such an infection at some
time.

Approximately fifty varieties of fungi can invade
human tissues. Fungi are larger than bacteria but still
visible only with the aid of a microscope. They are
classified into two groups: *dermatophytes,* close relatives
of household molds and mildew, and *yeasts,* cousins of
the organisms on which bakeries and breweries rely.

Most fungus infections are mild and chronic, often
ignored or unnoticed by the affected individual; but
infections may be quite itchy or painful and some may
lead to scarring. Infections are more common and
more flagrant in warm climates and during the summer
in temperate climates.

Dermatophytes and yeasts usually produce different
rashes, have their own favorite places on the body, and
respond to different medications. For these reasons we
deal with them separately — dermatophytes here, and
yeasts in Chapter 33. But beyond this basic grouping, it
is nearly impossible to identify from the clinical characteristics the species of fungus causing a given infec-

tion. The character of a fungus infection depends primarily on its location on the body and on the way in which the person's system reacts to the infection. A single organism may infect any area of the body. Conversely, fungal infection in a specified area can be due to any of several dozen species.

Athlete's foot (tinea pedis) is exceedingly common. It is unusual in childhood, but many adults have lived with it so long that they consider the mild scaling of their soles and the moist white skin between their toes to be normal. In its mild form, the infection seems harmless — at worst, it causes mild itching. However, in certain cases deep painful fissures subsequently form between the toes. These fissures may then be invaded by bacteria and lead to major infections. Moreover, once the fungus has a "foothold," it may spread to the groin, the hands, or other body areas. If the skin of the feet remains infected for a prolonged period, the toenails virtually always become infected as well. After this, the infection is much more difficult if not impossible to eradicate. Fungus-infected toenails are thickened, crumbly, and discolored. They frequently catch on socks or stockings. Fungi may also infect the fingernails.

Treatment of mild cases of athlete's foot is easy. Several antifungal sprays, powders, solutions, and creams are available without prescription in most drugstores. Tolnaftate (Tinactin®) is probably the most effective of these medications. Other excellent products are available but require a prescription from your doctor. It is worth noting that widely prescribed products such as Mycolog® are effective against yeast species of fungus but are useless in the treatment of dermatophyte infections. All of these medicines should be applied to the affected areas two or three times daily for

210

three or four weeks. An infection is not adequately treated until the skin appears completely normal for at least one week. Sprinkling an antifungal powder in shoes and socks helps destroy organisms that are shed from the feet and that otherwise form a reservoir for reinfection. Since fungi like warm, moist environments, sneakers and other occlusive shoes should be avoided.

Reinfection can be prevented by observing the above precautions and by using an antifungal powder on the feet once daily, especially in warm weather.

More severe infections, with oozing, crusting, and fissures between the toes require preliminary treatment in order for the above regimen to be effective. Add one teaspoon of table salt to one pint of tepid water. Soak the toes in a basin of this solution for fifteen minutes three or four times daily until the oozing has stopped, usually less than a week. After each soaking, pat the skin dry with a disposable towel and apply antifungal medication. *If at any time the back of the foot becomes swollen and tender or if red streaks appear, leading away from the area of the fungal infection, see your physician immediately.* These changes may indicate a secondary bacterial infection, a dangerous complication of athlete's foot.

If the toenails are involved, it is still worthwhile to treat infected areas of skin, but it is useless to apply creams or solutions to the nails. To restore the nails, a medication called *griseofulvin* must be taken in pill form for several months to a year. The cost of such treatment usually exceeds $300, and nearly half the time nail infection recurs within a year. If the expense and uncertainty are acceptable, however, consult a dermatologist. He or she can determine if nail abnormalities are indeed due to fungal infection (since psoriasis and other disorders can cause similar changes) and can prescribe the necessary medicine.

Jock itch (*tinea cruris*) is athlete's foot of the groin. The infection is most common in adult men who are either overweight or physically active and hence perspire heavily in the groin. The fungus usually involves the upper inner thighs primarily. The scrotum and anal area may also be infected. The rash is red, scaly, and often quite itchy. Treatment and prevention are the same as for athlete's foot. Because the fungus has usually spread from the feet, however, it is wise to medicate the toe web-spaces and soles as well as the groin, even if the skin there feels and looks normal. Loose cotton undergarments and other ways to prevent sweating in the groin are also helpful.

Ringworm (*tinea corporis*) differs from the other common fungal infections in that it occurs more often in children than in adults. Ringworm is named after its slightly itchy ring-shaped lesion, usually one or two inches in diameter, with a prominent scaly edge. The infection has nothing to do with worms. If there are only a few lesions, antifungal creams or solutions may be used. Extensive infections respond much better to a two- or three-week course of griseofulvin pills. In any case, *always* confirm the diagnosis of ringworm with your doctor before beginning treatment. If possible, see a dermatologist. Even experienced physicians frequently mistake eczema and other skin disorders for fungal infections.

The scalp is the most important area in which to detect and treat fungal infection promptly. Ringworm of the scalp (*tinea capitis*) is quite contagious and can produce areas of permanent hair loss if not treated early. Now fortunately uncommon, it was in former generations the scourge of school children. Until recently, no

212

safe, effective treatment existed. Fungi spread rapidly from child to child via contaminated barber's instruments, combs, and hats. Infected children might be expelled from school for extended periods or treated with poisons or later with dangerous doses of X-irradiation. Often the head was shaved as the first therapeutic measure. Control of tinea capitis is one of the minor miracles of modern medicine.

Fungal infection on the scalp usually begins as a small sore with broken and missing hairs, covered with a thick crust. Sometimes the skin itself is fairly normal, but all the hairs in the infected area are broken at the level of the scalp, creating a "black dot" appearance. In both cases the infected area gradually enlarges. Often bacterial infection confuses the picture. Diagnosis requires microscopic examination of skin scrapings and plucked hairs and appropriate fungal cultures. A dermatologist is usually better equipped for these procedures than are other physicians. Treatment of scalp ringworm involves special soaks and shampoos as well as griseofulvin pills. In promptly treated cases, there is no permanent damage, and even large boggy infections may eventually heal without scarring.

People wonder how they ever acquired a fungus infection in the first place. Public gymnasiums and pools are blamed for many cases of athlete's foot; advertisers proclaim household cleaners that kill germs causing athlete's foot. But it is really a matter of susceptibility: most people are constantly exposed to these fungi without developing an infection, while other people are repeatedly infected despite extreme precautions. Fungi are ubiquitous. The determining factor is not exposure, but rather the body's ability to fight fungus infection. People who have repeated or chronic fungal infections have a specific blind spot in their immune

213

defense systems. They are usually healthy in all other respects, but cannot prevent fungi from living and multiplying in the superficial layers of skin, in hair, or in nails. Such people may slightly reduce the likelihood of infection by avoiding warm, moist areas that are often heavily populated with fungi, such as locker-room floors and showers, but regular application of antifungal medication on their skin is a much more effective precaution. There is certainly no reason for a person not bothered by frequent fungus infections to avoid "high-risk" areas. Similarly, if one member of a family has athlete's foot, only those family members who have inherited the same susceptibility to fungi are likely to acquire the infection even if everyone is exposed to contaminated floors and towels. And susceptible family members are quite likely to become infected from a source outside their living quarters, even if they escape exposure at home.

The exception to this rule is ringworm in children. Perhaps because their immune defense systems are inexperienced and not fully mature, children frequently develop this infection if adequately exposed. Scalp ringworm seems especially contagious. Fortunately, ringworm ceases to be infectious after two or three days of appropriate treatment, even though it often takes two or three weeks for the lesions to disappear completely.

Ringworm illustrates the delicate balance between immunity and susceptibility in another way. Lesions begin as small spots where fungi invade the skin, but soon become rings with nearly normal skin in the center. This happens because the immune defenses of the body cannot quite catch up, and the most recently infected perimeter forms a ring around the healed center.

214

Fungus Infections

39
Shingles
(Herpes Zoster)

Shingles is the common name for *herpes zoster*, an infection caused by *varicella* virus, the same virus that causes chicken pox. Most people have chicken pox during childhood, but the disease may be mild, without a rash, so that the parents mistake the symptoms for a cold. After the acute infection, the virus is never completely eliminated from the body, but remains in an inactive state in nerve cells along the spinal cord. That may be the end of the story. However, in some people, the virus eventually reactivates, migrates to the skin, and causes shingles. The virus may wait in the nerve cell fifty or sixty years or may reappear much sooner.

Anyone who has had shingles can tell you it's an unpleasant business. Because nerves are involved, it is often quite painful. For days to weeks before the rash appears, there may be an aching or burning sensation in the area supplied by the infected nerve. This area is called a *dermatome*. Each dermatome begins at the spine and either wraps around one side of the face or body to the midline in front or extends down a limb. Depending on its location, the pain may be mistaken by pa-

215

tients and their doctors for migraine headaches, sciatica, or gallbladder disease, to name but a few. Eventually, the rash appears: warm red areas that quickly develop into clusters of weeping blisters. The pain and rash both follow the nerve pathway and so involve only one side of the body. Any dermatome may be affected, but those on the chest and upper face are favorites. Involvement of more than one dermatome at a time is rare. The infection may cause severe pain with only a few skin lesions, the rash may be very extensive and relatively painless, or both blisters and pain may be severe.

After a few weeks, the blisters dry up and heal. Especially in older people, however, pain may persist for many weeks or even months because of continued inflammation and sometimes scarring around the underlying nerve. An attack of shingles always ends eventually but may cause discomfort for months.

There are several facts worth knowing about shingles. First, the blister fluid contains varicella virus. Anyone who has not yet had chicken pox can get it by touching the fluid. For example, a grandparent with shingles should not hug small grandchildren until after all the blisters are dry and crusted and no longer infectious. If a member of the household is severely ill and unable to combat infections normally, he or she should be kept away from a person with shingles and should not handle the same kitchen or toilet articles. On the other hand, there is essentially no risk for healthy people who have had chicken pox, because they are immune to varicella virus. This includes almost everyone after the age of ten. In any case, the disease is contagious only while the blisters are weepy.

216   Second, treatment can help. Adequate relief of pain

often requires narcotics or other prescription medications. Your doctor may also recommend special soaks to hasten drying of the blisters and to prevent bacterial infection from beginning in the open sores. A teaspoon of table salt in a pint of tepid water may also be used. Wet a soft cloth in a basin of the solution and then place it gently over the blistered area for fifteen minutes every four to six hours until the skin is no longer weepy. In some cases, your doctor may prescribe medicine to prevent or reduce pain that may follow the skin eruption. If shingles affects the face, you should seek medical care immediately, because the eye itself may be damaged. An ophthalmologist or other physician capable of a complete eye examination should see you regularly until all danger is past. Prescription creams or eye drops may be necessary.

Why do people get shingles at a particular time in their lives? Shingles is a disease of partial immunity. The body recognizes the virus and can "contain" but not completely destroy it. Unless the balance is upset, the infection only rarely and briefly declares itself. Often shingles occurs at a time of stress, such as another illness or after surgery, when body defenses are lowered. It is often easy to confuse cause and effect, however. A person who believes he got shingles because he "sprained his back" gardening may have been experiencing the pain of shingles all along. Completely healthy, apparently unstressed people of any age may get shingles.

A person has chicken pox only once but may have shingles several times. Fortunately, this is unusual. Many people have shingles only once or twice in a lifetime and most people never have it. The only way to prevent shingles is never to have chicken pox, and trying to avoid this highly contagious childhood illness is risky because it is usually a mild disease in children but often a severe illness in susceptible adults. The average adult is better off having shingles than chicken pox.

Shingles (Herpes Zoster)

40
Hives
(Urticaria)

Hives are numerous weltlike extremely itchy skin lesions resembling large mosquito bites, each of which lasts less than a day and then disappears completely. Sometimes the eyes and lips also swell. In most cases, the entire process lasts only a few days. Hives is thought to be an allergic response to something the person ate or breathed or otherwise encountered, but often no culprit can be identified.

It can happen to anyone and is especially common in healthy young adults. A typical patient is a college student who, soon after a fancy seafood dinner, is covered with red welts and has to be taken to a nearby emergency room for relief of severe itching and sense of panic.

When hives are a manifestation of allergy, they may return with every exposure to the responsible substance. Seafood, tomatoes, and penicillin are frequent offenders. Such an allergy usually becomes apparent to the victim after a few attacks. For instance, hives occur within hours of eating clam chowder at a favorite restaurant, week after week. Substituting onion soup ends the problem. In such a case, testing in a doctor's office is not necessary to diagnose allergy to clams. Cure is accomplished by avoiding the allergen.

Often the problem is more complex. Hives seem to occur without unusual exposures or to persist for months, no matter how you alter your diet and household. In this situation, a physician can help by prescribing medicines that reduce both the itching and the tendency to form new hives. Sometimes an experienced physician can identify the responsible substance through detective work, consisting of careful questioning and intentional exposure to suspected foods or drugs. In some cases, blood tests or other laboratory investigations are necessary to exclude internal illness.

Hives are not contagious and in themselves not dangerous. If you are taking medication by mouth or by injection when the rash appears, discontinue the drug and consult your physician, since future allergic reactions to the substance may be more severe. If hives are not related to drug allergy and occur infrequently, there is no harm in "riding it out." The home treatments for itching suggested in Chapter 20 are often helpful. It is best to avoid aspirin during attacks, however, since this drug exacerbates hives in some people.

Hives (Urticaria)

41
Lupus Erythematosus

Many people are now acquainted with this once obscure and exotic disease. Systemic lupus erythematosus is rightfully feared by young women, who are its principal victims. Our discussion here will focus on the type of lupus that affects only the skin and will deal with some common misunderstandings and concerns expressed by patients.

Discoid lupus erythematosus (DLE) is the name for a specific type of skin lesion that begins as a raised, red, sometimes itchy area, and if untreated often leaves a scar. The appearance of the rash is classic: a dermatologist can recognize it immediately. In questionable cases, a biopsy virtually always permits diagnosis. Discoid lupus may occur anywhere on the body, at any age, in men or women. It is not rare. The face, mouth, ears, and scalp are most often involved.

Ninety-nine times out of one hundred, patients with DLE have only a skin disease. A few patients develop problems in other parts of the body either before or after DLE appears, but this is most unusual.

Patients with DLE often worry unnecessarily about the significance of their skin lesions. They fear that they have or will have *systemic* (generalized) *lupus erythematosus*. Systemic lupus erythematosus (SLE) is a potentially very serious condition that can affect the kidneys, lungs, liver, heart, brain, and other organs in addition to causing skin lesions.

Why do SLE and DLE have such similar names if they are not part of the same disease process? Many physicians regret this confusing terminology. The diseases have features in common but are certainly no more alike than, say, a cat and a lion — which, although members of the same family, leave very different kinds of injuries when attacking their victims.

Another concern of patients is the significance of "sun sensitivity." It is true that patients with systemic lupus erythematosus may develop rashes in light-exposed areas or become acutely ill after sunbathing; most patients with DLE also tend to develop lesions in sun-exposed areas. Neither of these problems is as common as simple sunburning, and only rarely does the rash of systemic lupus resemble sunburn. DLE never looks like a sunburn. If you sunburn easily, use a sunscreen, but don't worry that you have lupus.

People with DLE usually know it. The spots are easily detected by the patients themselves, tend not to disappear spontaneously, and, hence, prompt a visit to a doctor who, in most cases, can diagnose the condition.

If you have DLE, you should make regular visits to a qualified and concerned physician. This is terribly important. First, patients with DLE are at some risk, however small, of developing SLE: this can virtually always be detected early by a physician who is checking for the disease. Second, the lesions of DLE may be quite disfiguring and can usually be prevented or well-controlled by appropriate medical care, such as sun-

222

screens, topical steroid creams, or injection of steroids into the lesions to reduce inflammation, and in some cases, antimalarial drugs, which for unknown reasons are also beneficial.

42

When to See
Your Doctor
and What to Expect

There are three situations for which you should see your doctor: when something is wrong and you think it may be serious or need treatment, but you are not sure; when you know what's wrong and what to expect, and therefore wish to be treated; and, for certain people, as a routine check to be sure nothing is wrong.

Most people who have a rash or notice a mark on the skin for the first time belong to the first group. They think the bump on an arm is just a mole but want to be sure it isn't a cancer. This is a very legitimate reason to see a dermatologist. Usually the problem is not serious, and then the patient is reassured. Occasionally, the doctor determines that the condition is serious and does need treatment; then a proper course of action can be taken.

Patients with chronic skin diseases constitute the bulk of most dermatologists' practices. Here emphasis is on therapy, not diagnosis. Many common diseases such as eczema and psoriasis are incurable at present but very treatable. Patients with such conditions benefit from regular office or hospital visits in order to review their responses to the current medical regimen and to consider new treatments if they are not doing as well as hoped. It is a tragedy when patients deny themselves such help because "I know what's wrong" or because "you can't cure it." Since new therapies are constantly becoming available, repeated efforts to obtain effective treatment should be made over the years, no matter how bleak the prospects seemed in the past. Some people read extensively to find leads to new treatments for their disorders and contact their physicians if one is found. This is worthwhile but often discouraging, since magazines and newspaper articles are usually overly optimistic. It is also important to remember that some helpful new therapies are not adequately discussed in the news media. Research on your own cannot fully replace consultation with your doctor.

We hope that most people in the last category, those who need routine dermatologic examination, have been informed of this by their physicians. A large pigmented birthmark, for example, should be examined annually for the possibility of a tumor arising within it. Fair-skinned persons, especially if they have had lots of sun exposure, or people with a history of prior X-ray therapy for the skin, should see a dermatologist every year after the age of forty to check for the appearance of skin cancer. If you have already had one skin cancer, your chance of having another one is one in three each year! Only a trained eye can detect these lesions when they are very small and easiest to treat.

What can you reasonably expect from your doctor, once you have decided to see him? The answer to this question depends, of course, on your doctor. Many excellent internists, surgeons, pediatricians, and general practitioners know very little about diseases of the skin. If they are good doctors, they will tell you whether or not they can diagnose your problem. If they cannot, usually they will still be able to tell you if it is a potentially serious disorder and will refer you to an expert for further evaluation if necessary. If your general physician does know what you have, he may choose to begin your therapy himself or may wish to refer you to a dermatologist who is more familiar with the medications available and the most effective way in which to use them.

In many cases, it is advisable to see a dermatologist in the first place. This is especially true if you live near a large hospital or medical center or in a town that has a dermatologist.

A dermatologist is a doctor who has had at least three years of training in diseases of the skin, in addition to regular medical training. He is a specialist whose business it is to know about all disorders of the skin, no matter how rare, and about all their possible treatments. Consulting a dermatologist gives you the satisfaction of knowing what you have and how to deal with it as quickly as possible. It gives your own physician the advantage of being sure of your diagnosis and having access to a specialist colleague who can assist him with your future management. Your own physician will not consider it insulting if you seek a specialist's opinion. Inform him in advance, if convenient, and ask the dermatologist to send your doctor a letter summarizing the visit.

Now we may ask, what can you expect from the dermatologist? First, he can almost always identify your disorder. In the great majority of cases, he can do this just by looking at the skin lesions. Sometimes, he will need to scrape the surface of a lesion, very much as you would with your fingernail, and examine the

226

scrapings under a microscope for evidence of viral, bacterial, or fungal disease. This procedure can be done in a few minutes while you are still in the examining room. Less often, perhaps one time in fifty, he will need to do a skin biopsy before he can make a firm diagnosis. The biopsy itself is simple. The skin is numbed by a local injection of anesthetic and then a small plug of skin, approximately 1/6 inch across and 1/8 inch deep, is removed. The place where the skin was taken is covered by gauze and an adhesive strip bandage; sometimes one stitch is used to close the hole, but usually this is unnecessary. The biopsied skin is sent to a pathologist who cuts and stains it, then examines it under the microscope to detect certain cell types or cell patterns. The pathologist then sends a report of his findings back to the dermatologist, who correlates the microscopic findings with the clinical findings to assign the correct diagnosis. In some places, the dermatologist serves as his own pathologist. This whole process takes several days to a week, so the patient must either telephone or return for a second visit at that time. If the skin has been stitched, the suture can be removed then.

So, usually on the first visit, the dermatologist can diagnose your disorder. At times, a diagnosis — accompanied by an explanation of why, where, how, when, and for how long — is all you need. A person with occasional cold sores, for example, may be satisfied to know that he has a viral infection that is annoying but harmless, is briefly contagious for others, and will probably appear in the same place for a week or so several times during his lifetime.

Often, knowing the diagnosis is not enough. If the condition is harmless, it may still be terribly unattractive or uncomfortable. If it is not harmless, it must be

227

treated appropriately. Your dermatologist will explain the nature of the condition to you and answer your questions. If a number of therapeutic approaches are possible, he will tell you their pros and cons and recommend a specific treatment for you. In most cases, he will then prescribe or administer the treatment himself. Sometimes he will refer you to another specialist — for example, if major surgery or X-irradiation is necessary.

Many skin diseases are curable or self-limited. A patient with such a disorder will need to see the dermatologist only a few times. Unfortunately, a large number of skin diseases are chronic, neither curable nor self-limited. Whether the dermatologist sees such patients regularly or refers them to their general physicians depends on the severity of the disease, the type of treatment being used, and whether the patient has other illnesses.

Finally, can you expect your dermatologist to make you better? Yes. Almost always. Indeed, many physicians choose to enter the field of dermatology because their skills and treatments will have such a large impact on the health and happiness of their patients. In few medical specialties is it possible to alter the course of illness so often and so dramatically.

When to See Your Doctor and What to Expect

Index

abdomen, 56, 59, 61, 205
abrasions, 175
acids, 41, 140, 154–155, 169
acne, 119, 135–141; and black skin, 78; at various ages, 55, 58, 60; in pregnancy, 62; and soaps, 40, 42, 44
acute glomerulonephritis, 176
adhesive strip bandage, 128, 129–130, 227
adolescence, 40, 58–60; and black skin, 81; and cysts, 73; and dandruff, 173; and eczema, 159; and hair patterns, 112–113; and pityriasis alba, 79
adrenal glands, 32, 59, 147
adulthood, 61; and alopecia areata, 109; and black skin, 80, 81; and cysts, 73; and freckles, 86; and moles, 97; and seborrheic dermatitis, 173; and shingles, 218; and warts, 155
A-Fil®, 62
Africans, 22
Afro, 82
"age spots," 65, 86
aging, 5; and black skin, 82–83; and blood vessels, 72; control of, 65–66; and fair skin, 84, 86, 89; and hair loss, 105; and nails, 114; and sun exposure, 22, 39
alcohol: and acne, 137; in astringents, 46; and diaper rash, 58; and herpes simplex, 183; and itching, 125; and wounds, 129
allergic contact dermatitis, 45, 125, 164, 169–172
allergy: cleansing agents, 44, 45; contact dermatitis, 169–172; and eczema, 157, 159, 160, 171; hives, 219–220; in infancy,

54; to lice, 193; to medications, 50, 122, 125, 132, 186, 200; poison ivy, 164, 168; scabies, 195
alopecia areata, 109–110
Alpha-Keri®, 47
aluminum salt, 50
Americaine®, 186
American Indians, 7
amino acids, 35
amniotic fluid, 54
anagen phase, 29
androgen. See testosterone
anemia, 54
anesthesia, 154, 155, 186
animal nature, 4, 6, 10–11
ankles, 99
antibiotics: for acne, 78, 140, 141; of bacteria, 36; and body odor, 50; for boils, 179; and cysts, 73; for folliculitis, 177; for impetigo, 176; and pruritus ani, 123; for venereal diseases, 200, 201; for yeast infections, 188
antibodies, 37
anticancer drugs, 31
antihistamines: and eczema, 78, 80, 163; and itching, 125; in pregnancy, 63
antimalarial drugs, 223
antimetabolites, 148–149
antiperspirants, 47–51
antiseptic, 44, 50
anus: and bacteria, 36; and itching, 123–124; and jock itch, 212; and venereal diseases, 199, 203, 205; and venereal warts, 207
apocrine glands, 24, 48, 60

arms, 59, 79, 112, 119, 162, 206. *See also* underarms
arsenic, 94
Arta®, 62, 78
arthritis, 127, 145
Asians, 22, 112
aspirin, 132, 220
asthma, 157, 158–159
astringents, 45, 46, 137
athlete's foot, 47–48, 210–212, 213–214
atopic dermatitis, 157
atopic eczema, 157
"autoimmune" etiology, 100
autonomic nervous system, 15
Aveeno®, 125
Aveenol®, 125
axillae. *See* underarms
axillary sweat, 47–48

back, 19, 48, 57, 71, 96, 135
bacitracin, 130, 176, 179, 183
bacteria, 17; and acne, 135, 137, 138, 140; and athlete's foot, 209, 210, 211; and body odor, 48, 49–50; and eczema, 159; and folliculitis, 177; and impetigo, 175, 176; in infancy, 54, 56, 57; and ringworm, 213; on skin, 35, 36–37; in skin injuries, 129–134; and venereal disease, 200, 201–203, 204, 205; and washing, 40, 41, 43–44; and yeast infections, 188, 189
bacterial cultures, 200, 205
bacterial infection. *See* infection
baldness, 31, 32, 82–83, 105–111
Balnetar®, 163
Barrie, Sir James, 8
basal cell carcinoma, 93–96, 97
basal cells, 20, 21, 33
basement membrane, 27
bath oil, 47, 161
bathing: in adolescence, 60; and corns, 128; and eczema, 161, 162; and itching, 123, 125; normal skin care, 37, 40, 46–47, 48; and psoriasis, 146; and sunburn, 132
beard, 32, 59, 60, 156, 191; and black skin, 81–82
Beau's lines, 115–116
beauty, 3–8
beer, 51
Benoxyl®, 138
benzoyl peroxide, 138
Betadine®, 177
bidet, 47, 124
biopsy, 92, 98, 200, 203, 221, 227
birth control: devices and venereal disease, 199; pills, 111, 120, 136, 140, 189
birthmarks, 60, 69–71, 80, 97, 225
black skin, 22, 23, 71, 77–83, 95–96
blackheads, 135, 139
bleeding, 73, 97, 129, 130, 154, 156
blisters: of cold sores, 180–181, 182, 183; definition and care of, 129, 130–131; in eczema, 157, 159, 171; in genital herpes simplex, 185; in poison ivy, 166, 167; in scabies, 195; in shingles, 216, 217
Block-Out®, 85
blonds, 84, 104
blood, 11, 14, 16, 37, 143, 145, 202, 205; disease, 122
blood test, 179, 190, 200, 202, 203, 204, 205, 220
blood vessels, 18, 119–120; and dermis, 25; and eczema, 158; in fair skin, 86; in infancy, 53; malformations of, 69, 72–73; and nails, 33; in old age, 64; in pregnancy, 62; and seborrheic dermatitis, 174; in skin cancer, 93
blue eyes, 84
blunt dissection, 155
body odor, 43, 47–51, 58
boils, 177–179
bone marrow, 148
bowel movements, 47, 124
brain, 9, 13, 14, 22, 71, 121, 182; and syphilis, 203, 204; and systemic lupus, 222; tumors, 91, 95
Brasivol®, 137
breasts, 55, 59, 60, 95, 146, 189
bruises, 13, 64
BUF-PUF®, 137
burns, 14; on black skin, 78; and impetigo, 175; and psoriasis, 143, 146; treatment, 129, 130–132. *See also* sunburn
buttocks, 56, 59, 65–66, 71, 177, 195

calamine lotion, 167
callus, 21
cancer, 92, 94–95, 96, 122, 148, 187. *See also* skin cancer
Candida albicans, 188
candidiasis, 188
capillaries, 26–27, 72–73, 119
carbohydrates, 35
carbuncles, 177–179
catagen phase, 29
Caucasians, 7, 22, 71, 77, 112
cells. *See under specific names*
cervix, 187, 205
Chap Stick®, 75

melanocytes, 22; mongolian spots, 71; sex hormones, 55; skin diseases, 63; syphilis, 201
fever, 31, 132, 178, 181, 185, 203, 205
fibroblasts, 25–26
fingers, 33, 145, 167, 171, 195
folliculitis, 177
food, 10, 140, 160
Food and Drug Administration, 42
Food, Drug and Cosmetic Act, 49
forehead, 61, 139
Fostex®, 137
Fowler's solution, 94
freckles, 86
freezing, 72, 95, 154, 207
friction, 18
frostbite, 132–133
fruit juices, 51
fungi, 36, 40, 117, 123–124; infection, 209–214, 227
furuncles, 177–179

gametes, 149
garment nevus, 71
gauze pad, 130, 133, 167, 227
gelatin, 51, 115
gels, 137, 138, 146, 147
genital herpes simplex, 185–187
genitalia: and adolescence, 59; arousal, 16; and bacteria, 35, 48; and cold sores, 180; in infancy, 55, 56; and pigment loss, 99; pruritus vulvae, 124; psoriasis, 146; venereal diseases, 89, 185–187, 198, 202, 207
germs, 35, 129, 199
gloves, 76, 190
glycerin, 44
gonads, 59
gonococci, 204
gonorrhea, 197, 199–200, 204–206
gooseflesh, 28
griseofulvin, 211, 212, 214
groin, 144, 185, 189, 202, 210, 212
grouping, 6, 7
gynecologic examinations, 187

hair, 7; and acne, 139; in adolescence, 59–60; and bacteria, 37; and black skin, 81–82; braiding, 82; in childhood, 58; color, 32–33; curly, 32; and communication, 14, 16; and dandruff, 103–104; epidermal origin, 20, 24–25, 28–29; excess, 112–113; follicles, 27, 28–29, 30, 31–32, 34, 35, 109, 173, 177–178; folliculitis, 177; and fungal infections, 212–213; gray, 5, 104; growth, 3, 17,

29–32, 104; in infancy, 54–55; and lice, 191, 192, 193; loss, 32, 105–111; and moles, 70; in old age, 64; in pregnancy, 62; products for, 51; shaving, 5; transplantation, 107–108, 110; and venereal disease, 203; and vitiligo, 99
Halog®, 183
hammertoes, 127
hand eczema, 171–172
hands, 3; and athlete's foot, 210; and bacteria, 36, 37; and blood vessels, 119; and chapping, 75–76; and contact dermatitis, 169; and eczema, 158; and fair skin, 86; and frostbite, 33; in infancy, 53; in old age, 65; and poison ivy, 165; in pregnancy, 62; and skin cancer, 93; and venereal disease, 198, 206; washing of, 44; and yeast infections, 189, 190
hay fever, 157, 159
head, 28, 95, 107–109, 191–192, 193
hearing, 13
heart, 145, 204, 222
heat, 18; in infancy, 54; and itching, 123; and subcutaneous tissue, 27; and sunbathing, 89; and sweating, 48; and yeast infections, 188
hemangiomas, 69, 72–73
herbs, 51
heredity: and acne, 136; and baldness, 106–107; and eczema, 157; and excess hair, 112; and psoriasis, 143–144, 150; and skin cancer, 94; and subcutaneous tissue, 27; and warts, 153
herpes keratitis, 181–182
herpes progenitalis, 185–187
herpes simplex, 159, 180–184, 198
herpes virus hominis, 180, 185
herpes zoster, 215–218
Herplex®, 183
high blood pressure, 167
hirsutism, 112–113
hives, 219–220
hooves, 17, 20
hormones, 27; and acne, 136; in adolescence, 6, 58–60; and blood vessels, 120; in creams, 45; and excess hair, 112, 113; and hair, 31–32, 106–107, 111; in infancy, 54–55; in menopause, 64–65; in pregnancy, 6, 62; and psoriasis, 147
horns, 17, 20
hot flashes, 64
humidifier, 161
humidity, 18, 56, 75
hydrocortisone, 124, 174
hydrogen peroxide, 113, 130, 134
hydroquinone, 78

hyperpigmentation, 80, 81
hypnotism, 155

ice, 131
idoxuridine, 183
illness, 8; and cold sores, 181, 182; and
    dermatologists, 228; and hair, 31, 111;
    and nails, 34, 114, 115–116; and shin-
    gles, 217–218
immortality, 4–5
immune defense system, 37, 98, 100, 152,
    181, 189, 213–214, 217
impetigo, 159, 175–176
infants, 53–58; and cold sores, 182; and
    "cradle cap," 104; and eczema, 159, 160;
    and fair skin, 86; and genital herpes
    simplex, 187; and mongolian spots, 71;
    and seborrheic dermatitis, 173; and
    self, 9; and syphilis, 204; and touch-
    ing, 15; and yeast infections, 189
infection: and acne, 139, 141; and athlete's
    foot, 211; boils, 177–178; of cold sores,
    180–181, 182; in cysts, 73; and der-
    matologists, 227; and eczema, 159, 171;
    folliculitis, 177; fungus, 209–214, 227;
    and genital herpes simplex, 185–187;
    impetigo, 175–176; lice, 191, 193; and
    psoriasis, 144; pus, 26; and shingles,
    217; and skin injuries, 129, 133–134; ve-
    nereal disease, 200, 202, 204, 205, 206;
    and warts, 154, 156; yeast, 188–190, 198
infrared rays, 89
ingrown toenails, 117–118
injury: to black skin, 78–79, 81; to nails,
    115; and psoriasis, 143; to skin, 129–134
insect bites, 175
insecticide, 94
intertrigo, 56
intestines, 148, 188
intrauterine trauma, 69
iron, 114
irritant contact dermatitis, 157, 169
Italians, 112
itching, 121–126: and black skin, 78, 80,
    81; and discoid lupus, 221; and eczema,
    157, 158, 160–163, 171; and hives, 219;
    and fungus infections, 209, 210; jock
    itch, 212; and lice, 191–192, 193; and
    poison ivy, 167; in pregnancy, 63; and
    psoriasis, 144; and scabies, 195, 196;
    and seborrheic dermatitis, 173–174; and
    yeast infections, 188

Japanese bath, 46–47
jock itch, 212

keloids, 80–81

keratin, 20, 24, 33
keratinocytes, 20–21, 25, 26–27, 28, 32
keratolytics, 147, 148
Keri®, 44
kidney, 122, 176, 203, 222
knees, 99, 133, 143, 159
knuckles, 99

Lanacaine®, 132
lanugo hair, 29
leather, 25
legs, 59, 62, 96, 112, 153, 156, 206
lemon juice, 113
lentigo, 65
"leper complex," 12
leprosy, 12, 100, 143
lice, 191–194, 196, 198
lichenification, 124
Lidex®, 183
life-styles, 96
Lifebuoy®, 43
"light box," 146
light treatments, 184
linea nigra, 61
lips, 7, 28, 112; chapping, 75–76; cold
    sores, 181; contact dermatitis, 169;
    hives, 219; sun exposure, 88; warts, 154
lipstick, 75
liquid nitrogen, 95, 154, 207
liver, 91, 122, 148, 203, 222
"liver spot," 65
lotions: acne, 137, 138, 141, 183; and itch-
    ing, 125, 126; and lice, 193; and skin
    dryness, 44; as skin soil, 41; steroid,
    104, 147; sunscreen, 88; tanning, 87–88
Lowila®, 44
lung cancer, 96
lungs, 91, 182, 222
lunula, 33
lymph channels, 25
lymph nodes: and boils, 178: and cold
    sores, 181; and cysts, 73–74; and genital
    herpes simplex, 185; and lice, 191; and
    skin cancer, 98; and syphilis, 202
lymphoma, 122

Magic Shave®, 82
male pattern hair loss, 32, 106–107
males: and acne, 136; in adolescence, 59;
    and baldness, 32, 106–109; beard prob-
    lems, 81–82, 156, 191; body hair, 112;
    and genital herpes simplex, 185;
    pruritus ani, 123–124
malignant melanoma, 70–71, 93, 95–98
mammals, 17
manicure, 116

melanin, 21–22, 23, 32–33, 78
melanocytes, 21–23; and black skin, 77; and hair color, 32–33; and moles, 70; and mongolian spots, 71; in old age, 64, 65; and pigment loss, 99; and skin cancer, 95
melanocytic nevi, 69
melanosomes, 22
melasma, 61–62
menopause, 64–65
menstruation, 60, 136
menthol, 125, 132
methotrexate, 149
microorganisms, 19, 35–39, 40, 50
microscopic examinations, 92, 188, 200, 202, 205, 209, 213, 226–227
milia, 54–55
miliaria, 56
milk, 140
mineral oil, 104
mites, 35
moisturizers, 44, 45, 46, 76, 86, 122, 125, 161
moles, 69, 70–71, 97, 224
mongolian spots, 71
monilial intertrigo, 188–189
monilial paronychia, 116
moniliasis, 188–190
monobenzylether of hydroquinone, 79
Montagu, Ashley, 15
mosquito bites, 121
mothballs, 54
mouth: and cold sores, 180; and discoid lupus, 221; odors, 50; and pigment loss, 99; and venereal disease, 199, 203; yeast in, 189
Mycolog®, 189, 210
Mycostatin®, 189

nails, 17, 27, 28, 33–34, 114–118; and athlete's foot, 210, 211–212, 214; and bacteria, 37; and boils, 179; epidermal origin, 20, 24, 25; and environment, 31; in old age, 64; in pregnancy, 62; and psoriasis, 143, 144–145; and yeast infection, 189, 190
naphthalene, 54
napkin dermatitis, 56–58
nausea, 132, 140
neck, 3, 16, 72, 86, 95
Neisseria gonorrhoeae, 204
neomycin, 50
nerves, 13, 14, 25, 123, 181, 215, 216
nervous tension. See emotional stress
neural crest, 22
Neutrogena®, 44
nevus flammeus, 72

nipples, 27, 48, 61, 112
"nits," 191, 193
nodules, 195
Norway, 96
nose, 88, 119, 176, 179
nystatin, 189

obesity, 144, 177, 188, 212
oil glands. See sebaceous glands
"oil spots," 117
oils: and acne, 135, 136–137; in adolescence, 60; and bacteria, 36; and chapping, 75; and dandruff, 103; and eczema, 161; in infancy, 55; in old age, 64; poison ivy, 165; and seborrhea, 173–174; as skin soil, 41–42
ointments; antibacterial or antibiotic, 130, 131, 175, 183; and chapping, 76; and genital herpes simplex, 186; and psoriasis, 147; as skin soil, 41; steroid, 162; and sunburns, 132; zinc oxide, 58, 88
old age, 5, 63–66
onychomycosis, 117
opthalmologist, 182, 217
organic material, 48
Orientals, 7, 22, 71
oxygen, 26–27

Pabafilm®, 85
Pabagel®, 85
Pabanol®, 85, 184
pain, 14; boils, 178; frostbite, 133; fungus infection, 209, 210; genital herpes simplex, 186; gonorrhea, 205–206; hand eczema, 171; and itching, 121; puncture wounds, 130; shingles, 215–217; sunburn, 86, 132; and sweat, 48; venereal warts, 207
palms, 28, 47, 48, 50, 112, 144, 158, 165, 171, 203. See also hands
papular lichenification, 80
para-aminobenzoic acid (PABA), 87
parasitic infestations, 122
paste, 146
patch tests, 170
pathologist, 227
pelvic inflammatory disease, 205
penicillin, 160, 176, 200, 201
penis: in adolescence, 59; and genital herpes simplex, 185, 186; and scabies, 195; and subcutaneous tissue, 27; and venereal diseases, 199, 204, 205, 207
perfume, 44, 45, 49, 58
Persadox®, 138
perspiration. See sweat

petrolatum, 58, 76, 185
phaeomelanin, 32
phenol, 125, 132
pHisoHex®, 177
pigment, pigmentation, 4, 12, 21–23; in acne, 135; and black skin, 77–80; and freckles, 86; loss of (vitiligo), 79, 99–102; in pregnancy, 61; and skin aging, 39, 83; and sun exposure, 22, 86; and tanning, 22, 90. *See also* melanocytes
pimples: acne, 135–136, 139; in black skin, 78; folliculitis, 177; and rosacea, 119; and socialization, 11; of yeast infection, 189
pityriasis alba, 79
Piz Buin®, 85
plantar warts, 152, 154
plastic adhesive tape, 133
plastic surgeon, 141
plastic wraps, 76, 147, 162
podiatrists, 154, 155
podophyllin, 207
poison ivy, 121, 164–168, 169
pollens, as skin soil, 41
pollutants, environmental, 41
"port wine stain," 72
postinflammatory hyperpigmentation, 78
powders, 124, 125, 189, 210, 211
pregnancy, 61–63; acne, 136; birthmarks, 69; genital herpes simplex, 187; hair growth, 31, 62; itching, 122; nail growth, 34, 62; sex hormones, 6, 120; venereal disease, 201, 203, 204; yeast infections, 188
Premarin®, 124
pressure, 14, 18
PreSun®, 85, 184
prickly heat, 56, 57
prostate gland, 204
protein: collagen, 26, 45, 64, 87; in creams, 45; in fair skin, 87; and hair, 30, 51; keratin, 20, 24, 33; and nails, 33, 115
pruritus ani, 47, 123–124
pruritus vulvae, 47, 124
psoralen, 101, 150
psoriasis, 12, 142–151, 163, 211; in adolescence, 60; and "cradle cap," 104; and dermatologists, 224; and itching, 121–122, 123; and nails, 116, 117; in pregnancy, 62
puberty, 32, 48; and moles, 71; and sex hormones, 6, 55, 59, 136
pubic area, 32, 59, 112, 192
puncture wounds, 130
pumice stone, 128
pus, 26, 116, 178, 206
pustule, 136, 178
PUVA, 88

quaternary ammonium, 58

rashes, 11; on black skin, 81; contact dermatitis, 164, 169–171; and discoid lupus, 221, 222; in eczema, 157; and fungus infections, 209–212; and hives, 220; and itching, 121–122; and physician visits, 224; poison ivy, 165–168; and shingles, 216; in syphilis, 202–203
razor blade, 131, 178
redheads, 84
Reflecta®, 62
repigmentation, 101–102
resorcinol, 138
rheumatic fever, 175–176
Rhus toxicodendron. See Poison ivy
rickets, 22
ringworm, 94, 212–213
rosacea, 119–120
RVPABA®, 88

salicylic acid, 103, 128, 138, 147
Sarcoptes scabiei, 195
scab, 133
scabies, 195–196
scales, 17, 36, 103–104, 143, 147, 212
scaling, 53, 210
scalp: and bacteria, 36; and dandruff, 103–104; and discoid lupus, 221; and eczema, 159; and hair, 28, 30, 33; and hair loss, 105, 106, 108, 109, 111; in infancy, 55; and lice, 191; in old age, 64; and psoriasis, 143, 144, 147; ringworm, 94, 212–213; and seborrhea, 173; and venereal disease, 203
scars: acne, 137, 139, 141; on black skin, 78, 80–81; burn, 132; carbuncles, 178; and cold sores, 181; and collagen, 26; and discoid lupus, 221; and eczema, 159; and fungus infection, 209, 213; and gonorrhea, 204; and hemangiomas, 72; and impetigo, 176; and moles, 70; in old age, 64; and skin cancer, 95; and skin injuries, 130; and warts, 153, 154, 156, 208
scent gland, 24
scrapes, 129
scratches, 78, 143, 175
scratching, 123, 124–125, 144, 166, 191, 195; and eczema, 158–159, 160, 163
scrotum, 27, 59, 212
scurvy, 26
sebaceous glands: and acne, 135–137, 139; at various ages, 54, 55, 58, 60, 64; and bacteria, 36; and body odor, 49; and dermis, 27; epidermal origin, 24, 28

seborrhea, 173–174
seborrheic dermatitis, 104, 173
seborrheic keratosis, 65
sebum, 35, 36, 49, 135, 140, 173
self, 9–12
sensory function of skin, 13–16
sexual intercourse, 16; in adolescence, 60; and bidet, 47; and genital herpes simplex, 186–187; and lice, 192; in menopause, 64; and venereal diseases, 197–199, 201, 203, 207–208; and yeast infections, 190
sexuality, 5–6, 16, 27, 48, 197–198
shampoos, 51, 103–104, 193, 213
shaving, 5, 81–82, 113, 156, 179, 193
shin, 27, 144
shingles, 215–218
shoes, 117, 127, 211
showering. See bathing
silicone, 141
sitz baths, 186
skin cancer, 70, 91–98, 156; and black skin, 83; and cysts, 73; and dermatologists, 225; and moles, 70–71; and sun exposure, 22, 39, 84, 86–87, 92–97
skin diseases: attitudes toward, 11–12, 197; and dermatologists, 224–228. See also specific names
skin dyes, 101
skin fresheners, 46
skin soils, 40–41
skin toners, 86
skin tumors. See skin cancer
skin types, 84–90, 92, 93
sleep, 123, 137, 139, 161
smell, 13
smallpox, 159
soaps, 7, 41–44, 47, 50, 103; and acne, 137, 139; and boils, 179; and diaper rash, 57; and eczema, 158; and folliculitis, 177; and impetigo, 176; and seborrhea, 173; and skin injuries, 129, 134
socialization, 11
Solarcaine®, 132
soles, 47, 50, 112, 117, 144, 152, 171, 203, 212. See also feet
South America, 47
spices, 48
spider angiomas, 62
spinal cord, 13, 22–23, 71, 215
splint, 133
"spring tonics," 94
squamous cell carcinoma, 93–95, 96, 97
staphylococci, 36, 175, 177
starvation, 31, 114
steroid medications, 58, 79, 80, 82, 104, 110, 124, 131, 132, 147–148, 162–163,

166, 167, 174, 182, 183, 223
stomach, 148
"stork bite," 72
Stoxil®, 183
stratum corneum, 20–21, 25, 29, 33; and dermis, 27; and diaper rash, 57; and microorganisms, 36–37; and skin dyes, 101
strawberry hemangioma, 72–73
"strep throat," 144, 175–176
streptococci, 175–176
"stretch marks," 61, 63
striae, 61
sty, 177
subcutaneous tissue, 27, 64, 119
sugar, 188
sulfur, 103, 138
sunburn, 39, 46, 132; and acne, 138; and cold sores, 181, 183–184; and discoid lupus, 222; and fair skin, 84–86; and itching, 125; and pigment loss, 99; and psoriasis, 145; and skin cancer, 92
sun exposure: and acne, 138–139; and aging, 39, 65; and black skin, 82–83; and blood vessels, 119; and fair skin, 84–90, 225; in infancy, 54; and itching, 125; and melanin in melanocytes, 21–23; and psoriasis, 145–146; in pregnancy, 62; and skin cancer, 22, 39, 84, 86–87, 92–97; and skin dryness, 46; and sunburn, 86, 132; and systemic lupus, 222; and vitiligo, 101
sunlamp, 138, 146
sunscreens: need for, 66, 87–90, 94, 97, 100, 184, 222–223; in pregnancy, 62; table, 85
surgery: for corns, 128; and dermatologists, 228; and hemangiomas, 72; and keloids, 80; and shingles, 217; for skin cancer, 95, 97; and warts, 155
sweat, 14, 18; control of, 47–51; and eczema, 160; and germs, 35; in infancy, 56; and itching, 123; and makeup, 101; and odor, 43, 48, 49; in old age, 64; in pregnancy, 62; and sunscreens, 88; and washing, 40–41, 43
sweat glands, 17, 24–25, 27, 48, 55–56, 60, 64
swimming, 88, 101, 143
sycosis barbae, 81–82
synthetic material, 123
syphilis, 197, 199, 201–204
syphilitic chancre, 202
systemic lupus erythematosus, 222

tanning, 22, 23, 85, 87–88, 89–90, 92, 95, 96, 100, 125, 138

tar products, 104, 146–147, 148, 163
taste, 13
telangiectasia, 119–120
telogen effluvium, 111
telogen phase, 29
temperature, 14, 18; and blood vessels, 119; body, 24, 48; and eczema, 160; and frostbite, 132; and infancy, 53, 56; and psoriasis, 145; of skin, and bacteria, 37
testosterone, 31–32, 59, 106, 136
tetanus booster shot, 130
tetracycline, 120, 140
thighs, 56, 59, 177, 195, 212
throat, 176, 205
thrush, 189
thyroid: cancer, 94–95; disease, 100, 118, 122
Tinactin®, 210
tincture of iodine, 129
tinea capitis, 212–213
tinea corporis, 212
tinea cruris, 212
tinea pedis, 210–212
titanium oxide, 88
toenails, 33, 117, 211; ingrown, 117–118
toes, 127–128, 167, 210–212
toilet paper, 124
tolnaflate, 210
topical anesthetics, 125, 167
topical antiseptics, 134
touch, 13–14, 15–16
toupees, 107
tranquilizers, 125, 163
Treponema pallidum, 201
trichimonas, 124
trunk, 36, 159
Tucks®, 124
tumors. *See* skin cancer

Ubangis, 7
ulcers, 93, 167
ultraviolet light, 88, 89, 101, 146, 148, 150
underarms: bacteria in, 36; and deodorants, 48, 49; and hair, 32, 59, 112; and lice, 192; and poison ivy, 167
Updike, John, 142
urethra, 204
urination, 47, 124, 185, 186, 204
urine, 10, 11, 57, 204; tests, 179, 190
urticaria, 219–220
uterus, 61, 62, 205
UV-A, 150
Uval®, 88

vaccinations, 98, 159–160, 184
vagina: in adolescence, 59; and bacteria, 35, 54; in menopause, 64; in pregnancy, 62; and venereal diseases, 199, 204, 207; yeast infections of, 124, 140, 189
varicella, 215, 216
varicose veins, 62
Vaseline®, 58
vegetable shortening, 161
Vel®, 43
vellus hairs, 32, 55
venereal diseases, 60, 185–186, 195–196, 197–206; warts, 207–208
vernix caseosa, 54
vinegar douche, 140
viruses: and bacteria, 36; and diagnosis, 227; herpes simplex, 180–187; shingles, 215–218; warts, 152, 156, 207–208
vision, 13
vitamin C, 26
vitamin D, 22
vitamin E creams, 45
vitamins, 7, 35, 45
vitiligo, 79, 99–102
vomitus, 10, 11
vulva, 124–125, 203

washing, 40–47, 48; and acne, 137; and chapping, 75; and diaper rash, 57; of hair, 51; and poison ivy, 165; and pruritus ani, 124; and pruritus vulvae, 124; and seborrhea, 173; and sunscreens, 88
warts, 152–156; venereal, 198, 199, 207–208
water: and boils, 178; in body, 11, 18–19; and chapping, 75; and dermis, 25; and germs, 35; and impetigo, 176; and infancy, 54; loss, 46, 47; and old age, 64; and sexual intercourse, 47; and shingles, 217; and skin injuries, 129–130, 131–134; and skin soils, 41–42, 46; and sweating, 48; and yeast infections, 116, 189–190
weather: and chapping, 75; and eczema, 160–161; and hair growth, 31; and old age, 64; and sun damage, 87, 89, 92, 96
white blood cells, 136
whiteheads, 135
wigs, 107, 110
windburn, 39
witch hazel, 124
wrinkling, 5, 39, 65, 86
wrists, 195

X rays, 31, 72, 81, 94–95, 213, 215, 228